Hèla Ben Jmaà

Heart tumors: Diagnosis and treatment

Hèla Ben Jmaà

Heart tumors: Diagnosis and treatment

Heart tumors

ScienciaScripts

Imprint

Cover image: www.ingimage.com

This book is a translation from the original published under ISBN 978-620-6-71878-9.

Publisher:
Sciencia Scripts
is a trademark of
Dodo Books Indian Ocean Ltd. and OmniScriptum S.R.L publishing group

120 High Road, East Finchley, London, N2 9ED, United Kingdom
Str. Armeneasca 28/1, office 1, Chisinau MD-2012, Republic of Moldova, Europe
Printed at: see last page
ISBN: 978-620-8-04045-1

TABLE OF CONTENTS

ABBREVIATIONS :

ACE: Embryonic Carcino Antigen

DNA: Deoxyribonucleic acid

C3: Complement 3

CA 125: Carcinoid Antigen 125

ECC: Extracorporeal Circulation

CIA: Interaural communication

IVC: Ventricular septal defect

Cm: Centimeter

CMG: Cardiomegaly

CRP: C Reactive Protein

DPN: Paroxysmal nocturnal dyspnea

ECG: Electrocardiogram

TEE: Transesophageal ultrasound

TTE: Trans-thoracic ultrasound

FM: Foyer Mitral

Gr: Gramme

Gy : Gray

ICD: Right heart failure

ICG: Congestive heart failure

MI: Myocardial Infarction

Ig G: Immunoglobulin G

IL 6: Interleukin 6

MI: Mitral insufficiency

MRI: Magnetic Resonance Imaging

Mm: Millimeter

MPS: Mucopolysaccharide

NS: Our series

NSE: Neurone Specific Enolase

OD: Right earpiece

OG: Left earpiece

OS: Osteosarcoma

PNE: Polynuclear Eosinophils

PS100: Protein S100

ITP: Inflammatory pseudotumor

RD: Diastolic bearing

MVR: Mitral valve replacement

SIA: Interaural Septum

IVS: Interventricular Septum

SS: Systolic sigh

CT: computed tomography

VD: Right ventricle

LV: Left ventricle

HIV: Human Immunodeficiency Virus

VM: Mitral valve

VS: Sedimentation rate

I- Introduction :

Cardiac tumors are those that develop from the various elements of the endocardium, myocardium and pericardium.

Metastases have a higher incidence than primary tumors. As far as primary tumors are concerned, myxoma is the most frequent tumor in the cavitary region, in contrast to the valvular location, where fibroelastoma predominates [1].

Clinical symptoms are polymorphous. It depends more on the location of the tumor than on its size. A large tumor infiltrating the cardiac muscle may be clinically asymptomatic, while a small tumor located in the valvular endocardium may impede blood flow and have a noisy clinical expression.

Diagnosis of these tumors is currently facilitated by non-invasive imaging techniques, in particular echocardiography.

The development of cardiac excision and reconstruction surgery has transformed this pathology into a curable condition.

II- History :

Tumors of the heart have long been recognized, as far back as Columbus's autopsy of Cardinal Gambara in 1559 [2, 3].

In the 17th century, Bartoletti and Piscini [2] introduced the term "polyp" of the heart to designate all the masses that can be found inside the heart, by analogy with uterine and nasal polyps.

In 1809, Burns [2] described a pedunculated tumor of the OD, engaged with the tricuspid valve and the VD. In 1843, De Puisaye [2] described a poly-lobed, grape-like, gelatinous, soft, pedunculated tumor of the OG in the region of the foramen ovale, while protruding into the LV through the mitral valve.

In 1945, Mahaim's [2] work on tumors of the heart contributed to the development of this chapter of cardiac pathology and to the clarification of ideas on surgical therapeutics. In 1947, he suggested angiography for patients with suspected cardiac tumors.

The advent of angiocardiography has been of major importance in the diagnosis of cardiac tumors in living subjects. It enabled the diagnosis of cardiac myxoma for the first time by Golberg and colleagues [4, 3] in 1952.

In 1954, Crafoord [5] performed the first surgical resection of an OG myxoma under CEC. In 1959, Effert and Domanig [6] suspected the value of echocardiography in the diagnosis of cardiac tumors.

In 1960, Cooley [7] described the first resection of the AIS and Franfenfeld reported the first cure of a bi-auricular myxoma [7].

Echocardiography, introduced in 1968 by Shattenberg [8, 3], provided the first echocardiographic diagnosis of atrial myxoma. Since then, it has been considered the method of choice for the early diagnosis of cardiac tumors and for monitoring their progress after surgical resection.

III- Epidemiology :

1- Frequency :

Primary tumors of the heart are rare. Their incidence ranges from 0.001% to 0.33% [9, 10, 11]. They are dominated by benign myxomas, which account for around 50% of all primary tumors of the heart, and are most often sporadic, although familial forms associating extra-cardiac lesions are described in 5% of cases [12].

Lipomas account for 8-12% of all primary cardiac tumours [13]. Inflammatory pseudotumors of the heart are extremely rare benign lesions of undetermined etiology. Their true incidence is unknown [14].
Rhabdomyomas are rare congenital tumors that preferentially affect children; they account for three quarters of neonatal cardiac tumors [14]. In more than half of cases, they are part of a phacomatosis: tuberous sclerosis of Bourneville [14]. After rhabdomyomas, fibromas are the second most common cavitary congenital tumor in children. Hemangiomas are benign vascular tumors that account for less than 2% of cardiac tumors [15]. They are often isolated, but may be associated with cutaneous hemangiomas, hepatic hemangiomas or Kasabach-Merritt syndrome (multiple hemangiomas, thrombocytopenia and coagulation disorders) [14].

Primary malignant tumors are rare, accounting for 25% of all primary tumors. The majority are sarcomas [59, 156]. Secondary tumors are 20 to 40 times more frequent than primary tumors [16]. Sarcomas account for 95% of primary cardiac malignancies.

The most common histological types are angiosarcomas (37%), undifferentiated sarcomas (24%), rhabdomyosarcomas (20-30%), fibrosarcomas (10-15%), leiomyosarcomas (8-9%) and osteosarcomas (3-9%) [9]. Liposarcoma is a very rare entity among primary sarcomas. Malignant histiocytofibroma is the most common adult soft-tissue sarcoma, but is extremely rare in the heart [17].

Lymphomas account for 5% of primary malignant tumours of the heart [18, 19]. Their incidence is increasing due to the rising rate of Epstein Barr virus and HIV infection in immunocompromised patients, and is also higher after heart transplantation [20]. Almost all cases are non-Hodgkin's type B malignant lymphomas.

Tawarian mesothelioma is an exceptional, small tumor localized in the atrioventricular node [14].

Primary tumors that metastasize to the heart are divided into three groups in order of frequency [9] :

- Those with a high incidence of metastasis: melanoma and bronchopulmonary cancers.

- Those at intermediate risk of metastasis: carcinomas of the liver, stomach, colon, rectum, ovaries, thyroid gland, esophagus, breast, lymphomas and leukemias.

- Those with a low risk of metastasis: this group is represented by the rest of the malignant tumors.

Although cardiac metastases are much more common than primary neoplasia, no cases were encountered in our patient group.

Papillary fibroelastomas have an estimated frequency of 0.0017 to 0.33% in autopsy series [21]. They account for 7% of benign tumours of the heart and are the most common valvular tumour [22]. Valvular localization of myxomas is extremely rare. Cardiac metastases are rarely valvular.

Pericardial hemangiomas have a frequency comparable to that of intracavitary hemangiomas. Benign teratomas are the most common pericardial tumor in children and infants. Primary pericardial tumors are rare. Mesotheliomas account for 50% of these tumors and 0.0022% of all cardiac tumors [23]. They are often associated with pleural localization. Pericardial lymphomas are most often an extension of cavitary lymphomas. Pericardial metastases are essentially lymphomas.

The respective frequencies of the different histological types of primary cardiac tumours are shown in Table I [22, 7, 13, 15, 23, 19] :

Table I: Frequency of the most frequent histological types of cardiac tumors.

	Location cavitary	***Location valvular***	***Location pericardial***
myxoma	62,25 %	Very rare	unknown
lipoma	8 à 12 %	Very rare	unknown
PTI	unknown	exceptional	unknown
hemangioma	0,06 %	exceptional	0,06 %
sarcoma	23,75 %	exceptional	rare
lymphoma	1,3 %	exceptional	rare
fibroelastoma	Very rare	5,25 %	unknown
mesothelioma	exceptional	exceptional	0,0022 %

2- Terrain :

Ninety percent of myxoma patients are between 30 and 60 years of age [24]. The average age is 50 [25]. Familial forms are seen in younger subjects. The majority of published series show a predominance of females, with a sex ratio of up to 0.33 [26, 27].

Lipomas and lipomatous hypertrophy of the IAT preferentially affect elderly subjects, with an average age of 70 [14]. There is no gender predilection.

Inflammatory pseudotumors (ITPs) are most common in children. They are rare in adults [28]. Li et al [29] published 7 cases affecting children aged between 4 months and 17 years. Coffin et al [30] also described 84 extra-pulmonary ITPs with a mean age of 12 years. There was no gender predilection.

Rhabdomyomas are the most common cardiac tumour in the paediatric population [31]. They account for 65% of primary cardiac tumors in infants. Cardiac fibromas are congenital tumors affecting children, a third of whom are under one year of age. They have no gender predilection.

Hemangiomas occur at an average age of 43 years. Their frequency is higher in men than in women [24]. Sarcomas occur mainly between the third and fifth decades of life, and range from 1 to 76 years of age.

In adults, angiosarcoma is the most common histological type. In children, these tumors are rare and dominated by rhabdomyosarcoma, followed by fibrosarcoma and malignant teratoma.

The average age at diagnosis of leiomyosarcomas is between 40 and 50 years, compared with 47 years for liposarcomas and undifferentiated sarcomas. They are predominantly male, with a sex ratio of between 2 and 3 [32].

The average age of patients with primary cardiac lymphoma is 38 years. There is a slight male predominance [24]. Cardiac metastases predominate in subjects in the sixth or seventh decade of life. The sex ratio is close to 1.

Fibroelastomas affect all age groups from the neonatal period to the tenth decade of life, but predominate in adults. The average age is 60. The sex ratio is close to 1 [33].

Valvular cardiac metastases mainly affect elderly subjects. The average age of onset of pericardial mesotheliomas is 46 years, with extremes ranging from 2 to 78 years. Teratomas are fetal tumours, diagnosed in over 80% of cases during pregnancy [34].

Table II: Field data from the literature [33, 28, 25, 32].

	Average age	Sex ratio	Average age
Myxoma	50	0,33	54
Fibroelastoma	60	1	37
PTI	12	1	31
Neurofibrosarcoma	50	< 1	17

3- Location:

The left atrium accounts for 75% to 90% of myxoma locations [35, 36, 7, 37, 38]. Implantation occurs mainly in the SIA, in the fossa ovale or at its margins. This predilection is explained by the fact that the fossa ovale is the site of elective sequestration of the multipotent embryonic cells that make up the myxoid tissue. They can also be inserted on the anterior and posterior surfaces of the atrium or in the left auricle.

15% to 20% of myxomas are located in the right auricle, particularly around the fossa ovale [36, 7]. More rarely, the insertion occurs near the opening of a vena cava or on the posterior wall [39, 35].

Ventricular forms are rare, and are mainly seen in young subjects. The frequency of left ventricular forms is estimated at between 2.5 and 4% of myxomas [40, 41, 42], and that of right ventricular forms at between 2 and 4% [43]. Multiple forms in the same chamber or in several heart chambers at the same time are possible, and are most often familial [43]. In a large series of 123 myxoma cases, Goswami et al [44] described only two cases of multiple myxoma localization in the right heart.

IV- Clinical study:

1- Circumstances of discovery :

Cardiac tumors are characterized by a high degree of clinical polymorphism, which can lead to delayed diagnosis. Clinical manifestations are determined by tumor location, size and mobility, rather than histological type. In the case of left-sided cardiac localization, symptoms are also conditioned by the tumor's relationship to the mitral orifice, given the impediment it causes to atrial emptying.

Exertional dyspnea is the most frequent symptom. The frequencies reported in the literature vary from 54 to 90% [37, 42].

Paroxysmal nocturnal dyspnea and acute pulmonary edema may be observed. These paroxysmal attacks are usually associated with tumor entrapment in the mitral orifice or obstruction of the proximal pulmonary veins. They may also be associated with massive pulmonary embolism or compressive neoplastic pericardial effusion [45].

True syncope is rare. They may be the only mode of expression of a mobile myxoma of the OG due to tumour enclosure in the mitral orifice. These syncopations usually occur with changes in position and are related to the abrupt drop in cardiac output when the tumour becomes enclosed [46]. Postural syndrome may also be manifested by lipothymia or its equivalents (visual blur, bright spots in front of the eyes).

Chest pain occurs in 10-20% of myxoma cases. They may be related to pericarditis or pulmonary embolism, or represent an angina attack or MI related to obstruction of a coronary ostium by an emboligenic tumor (often a papillary fibroelastoma) [14].

Hemoptysis is most often moderate, and is associated with tumoral pulmonary embolism or pulmonary metastasis of cardiac sarcoma or lymphoma.

Peripheral edema is a symptom of right ventricular failure. They are frequently observed in right atrial tumors impeding tricuspid valve kinetics [47]. Limb ischemia may be the consequence of peripheral embolism [48]. Dysphonia is a rare clinical manifestation whose presence reflects an advanced stage of the disease with distant metastases. Cyanosis is mainly seen in infants with congenital tumors.

Heart tumors can be revealed by other symptoms such as dry cough and palpitations.

General signs are frequently associated with myxoma, ITP, sarcoma and cardiac metastases. These general manifestations are often misleading, leading to errors and delays in diagnosis.

The signs described in the literature are numerous and varied. They include fever, altered general condition, arthralgias and myalgias, and more rarely skin lesions (erythema, papules, petechiae) or Raynaud's syndrome.

2- Physical examination :

The most important physical sign is an auscultatory abnormality whose modification according to the patient's position testifies to the tumor's mobility during the cardiac cycle.

2- 1- Left heart tumors :

In the case of OG tumors, an impression of B1 splitting may be noted, due to the hearing of the tumor's sudden expulsion from the ventricle.

Another interesting auscultatory feature is the tumor plop at the onset of ventricular diastole. This sound occurs after aortic closure and presents as a false mitral opening snap [49, 50].

Other auscultatory abnormalities may suggest mitral narrowing or disease, or more rarely mitral insufficiency.

A murmur of functional tricuspid insufficiency may be noted.

2- 2- Right heart tumors [49, 50, 51]:

In the case of OD tumours, auscultation reveals a diastolic, xiphoid murmur in 65% of cases, attesting to impaired atrial emptying. Systolic murmurs of tricuspid insufficiency are less frequent. In 9% of cases, auscultation remains normal.

Right ventricular localization is manifested auscultatorially by a left latero-sternal systolic ejection murmur, with or without signs of right ventricular failure pointing to the diagnosis of pulmonary narrowing.

Other auscultatory signs that may be present are gallop sounds in heart failure, and pericardial friction and muffled heart sounds in pericardial effusion.

V- Additional tests :

The aim of these examinations is to make a positive diagnosis of the cardiac tumor, suspect its benign or malignant nature, assess its locoregional extension and monitor its post-therapeutic evolution.

1- Chest X-ray [52, 37, 38]:

Chest radiography lacks specificity in tumor pathology. It may be normal or show abnormalities:

- A mitral silhouette in the case of tumors that narrow the mitral orifice and lead to progressive dilatation of the OG.
- Pulmonary arterial dilatation with vascular redistribution to the upper lobes.
- Increased cardiac silhouette due to pericardial effusion or CMG.
- Mediastinal opacity
- Pleural effusion resulting from heart failure or the presence of a primary or secondary lung tumour [49, 53].
- Images of costal osteolysis or pulmonary opacities [54].

2- Electrocardiogram :

ECG changes occur in 75% of cardiac tumors [49, 50, 55].

Electrical signs are often non-specific. The following may be observed:

- Atrial fibrillation or flutter
- Ventricular rhythm disorders
- Atrioventricular and interventricular conduction disorders due to invasion of conduction tissue
- Signs of atrial or left ventricular hypertrophy were found in 53% of OG myxomas in Peters' series [56].
- Right ventricular hypertrophy and right axial deviation
- Disturbances in myocardial repolarization or a Q wave associated with coronary embolism
- Microvoltage or electrical alternation may accompany pericarditis

- An enlarged P wave with a double hump appearance, biphasic P wave with initial broad positivity followed by narrow negativity called *dome and dip* very characteristic of atrial septal hypertrophy [14].

3- Echocardiography:

Echocardiography has established itself as the technique of choice for diagnosing cardiac tumours. It has completely supplanted selective angiocardiography due to its non-invasive nature [57].

3- 1- ETT :

Because it is simple, inexpensive and non-invasive, TTE is now the first-line examination for any patient suspected of having a cardiac tumour. It is recognized by all authors [58, 59] as being highly effective for positive diagnosis and for studying the morphological characteristics of the tumour.

It specifies the tumor's size, shape, insertion base and consistency, and explores the other cavities for possible multiple synchronous localizations [60]. It also looks for stenosis or valvular regurgitation of tumoral origin.

It can show pericardial effusion, guide its drainage and guide percutaneous biopsy [61, 62].

However, this technique can be compromised by :

- False positives (embryonic remnants, localized ventricular parietal hypertrophy, thrombi, vegetations and artifacts).

- False negatives in the case of poor ultrasound windows or small tumors.

The typical myxoma appears on two-dimensional ultrasonography as a mass, often homogeneous, with regular contours, implanted on the SIA near the fossa ovale by a long pedicle. This more or less voluminous mass is animated by to-and-fro movements, sometimes with diastolic wedging into the mitral orifice or the LV (photo no. 1):

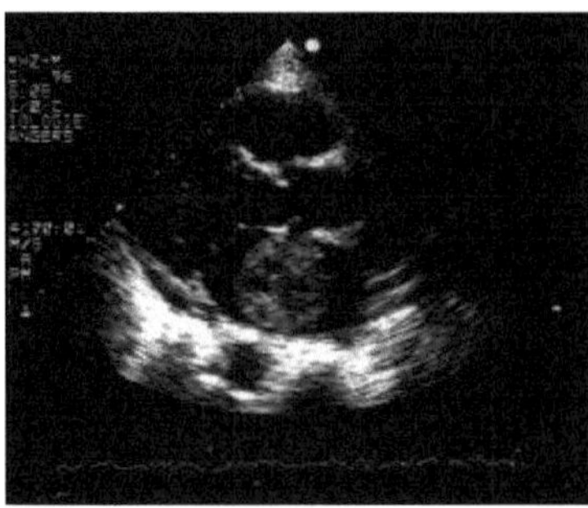

Photo 1: Two-dimensional echocardiography in longitudinal section of an OG myxoma prolapsing into the LV in diastole [14].

Non-prolapsing myxoma, sometimes unusually located at the bottom or top of the OG, is more difficult to diagnose. In such cases, TEE is of definite help.

On TTE, the lipoma appears as a well-circumscribed, hyperechogenic, cavitary mass [63]. Lipomatous hypertrophy of the AIS presents as a characteristic pathognomonic "dumbbell" or "diabolo" appearance of the AIS (septal thickness greater than 15 mm).

In the case of rhabdomyomas, TTE reveals homogeneous, hyperechoic nodules in the ventricular (photo no. 2) or septal walls, sometimes protruding into the heart chambers.

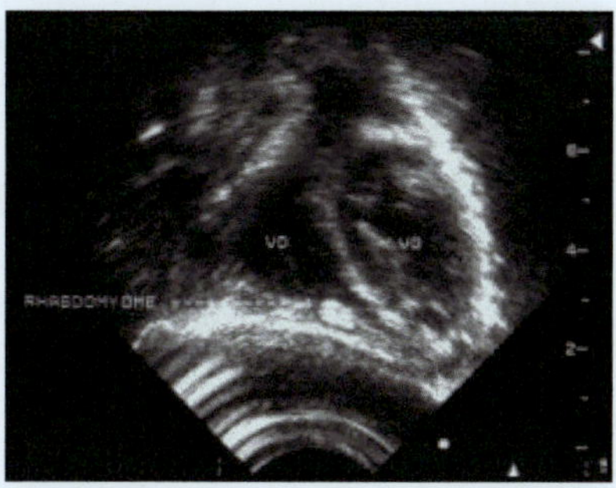

Photo 2: Rhabdomyoma appearing as a hyperechoic nodule in the right ventricular wall, protruding into the right ventricular cavity [14].

The fibroma appears on TTE as a single, hyper-echogenic, well-limited nodular mass embedded in the myocardial wall. In some cases, its echogenicity is close to that of normal myocardium. In these cases, MRI is the diagnostic tool.

The malignant nature of the tumour is suspected on TTE in the event of invasion of the inferior vena cava or parietal infiltration [14].

Ultrasound diagnosis of fibroelastomas is not always easy. It is essential to rule out the presence of vegetation associated with infective endocarditis. Fibroelastomas are small masses (often < 1.5 cm), often pedunculated, flapping and mobile, appended or attached to valvular tissue, most often localized on the atrial side when located on atrioventricular valves, but without a predilection for sigmoid valves. They are rarely associated with valvular dysfunction, despite the high frequency of localization on the valvular endocardium.

Pericardial tumors are masses are suspicious of malignancy if they are rounded and sessile or oblong, and if they are associated with pericardial effusion [14]. Ultrasound can be used to guide pericardial puncture and biopsy.

Table III compares the ultrasound characteristics of the histological types of tumors published in the literature.

Table III: Sonographic characteristics of cardiac tumors [14].

	Fibroelastoma		PTI	Neurofibrosarcoma
Size	Variable	< 1.5 cm	Variable	Large size
Echostructure	Hyper-echogenic	Hyper-echogenic	Hypoechoic	Heterogeneous
Mobility	mobile	Mobile	Fixed	Fixed
Insertion	Inter-auricular septum	Valvular endocardium	No seat preference	Invades all tunics

3- 2- OCT:

TEE has become an indispensable adjunct to the diagnostic strategy for cardiac tumours. Its greater sensitivity has been clearly demonstrated, particularly for the detection of hypodense tumours, tumours of the roof of the OG, multiple forms and in cases of poor patient echogenicity [58, 59]. It provides the surgeon with information on the existence or absence of adhesions between the tumour and the valvular structures. It also determines the site of attachment of the tumour, its size, the existence or absence of adherent thrombi and extension, notably through the fossa ovale; and estimates valve function. It is more discriminating than CT or MRI for lesions smaller than one cm.

Elements in favor of malignancy are reduced mobility, myocardial infiltration, broad base of implantation and more heterogeneous appearance with echogenic surfaces of varying degree.

TEE is similarly superior to TTE for the evaluation of right atrial myxomas, as it allows better visualization of both atria and the septum [59].

In a study of 13 myxomas comparing the respective merits of TTE and TEE, Zamorano [64] found that multiple locations were unrecognized on TTE and that the site of implantation was specified 9 times out of 13 by TTE and in all cases by TEE.

It is also useful intraoperatively to assess the outcome of any valve replacement. These observations support the superiority of TEE over TTE.

3- 3- 3-dimensional TEE [65]:

Recently, three-dimensional dynamic TEE has been introduced as a new diagnostic approach. It can give accurate spatial information about the shape and surface of masses, valve invasion; and study dynamic anatomy in real time.

3- 4- Intracardiac **ultrasound [66]:**

Biopsy of a right heart mass can be guided by intracardiac ultrasound. The probe is inserted through the femoral vein to the DO, and allows multiple biopsies of the mass to be guided.

3-5- Antenatal ultrasound :

Antenatal ultrasound is useful for the in-utero diagnosis of congenital tumors in the fetus [67].

4- Computed tomography :

It visualizes the size and density of the mass [68], tumor calcifications, and detects any fatty component of the tumor suggesting its nature (lipoma, liposarcoma).

It provides the necessary information on the invasion of adjacent structures, the presence of pleural effusion, mediastinal adenopathies and pulmonary metastases. It can also be used to study large vessels and the chest wall. It is also useful for differential diagnosis with other cardiac masses, notably thrombi.

But CT is still inferior to echocardiography in detecting and studying small moving structures such as valves.

5- MRI [14]:

Given the perfect spatial resolution of the endocardium and epicardium in MRI, and the possibility of multiplying incidences, the anatomical relationships of cardiac masses are perfectly established.

The use of both T1 and T2 offers a degree of tissue characterization that is enhanced by contrast agents, accentuating the heterogeneous appearance of malignant tumors.

MRI is therefore a reliable technique for the positive diagnosis of cardiac masses, specifying their relationship, mobility, size and location. It also specifies its mediastinal extension. MRI is more effective and more specific than ultrasound in differentiating an endo-luminal tumor from a thrombus. Cine-MRI enables dynamic visualization of tumor movements, thanks to synchronization of measurements with the ECG.

When in doubt about a malignant tumor, certain criteria are suspect:

- Poorly defined, polylobed appearance of the cardiac mass
- Invasion of large blood vessels
- Hemorrhagic pericardial effusion
- Heterogeneous mass signal after gadolinium injection
- Sometimes only T1 hypersignal without individualized tumor, associated with localized thickening of the myocardial wall.

It enables post-therapeutic monitoring of malignant cardiac lesions. This technique is the method of choice for assessing cerebral complications of emboligenic tumors, even in the absence of neurological signs [69].

6- Angiography:

Thanks to the precision of the information provided by ultrasound, angiography is no longer an essential part of the pre-operative work-up.

Angiocardiography visualizes the tumor as an intracavitary lacuna, assesses valvular function and detects any associated abnormalities in the large vessels. Right heart catheterization measures the pressure increase upstream of the tumor and the trans-tumoral pressure gradient.

7- Coronary angiography :

Coronary angiography is indicated for patients over 40 and for those with risk factors for atherosclerosis.

In some cases of myxoma, there is a characteristic neo-vascularization [70, 71]. This anatomical peculiarity explains some false-negative ultrasound findings, as the echogenicity of the tumour decreases and becomes similar to that of blood. Diagnosis is thus facilitated by coronary angiography.

Coronary angiography can also objectify coronary emboli [14]. However, angiography and cardiac catheterization can have false positives and false negatives, and run the risk of mobilizing the tumor during probe passage or contrast injection.

8- Biology :

Certain biological disturbances may be observed in patients with cardiac tumors. Their etiology is not clearly established. Some authors believe they are the consequence of tumor fragments passing into the general circulation, while others place them in the context of paraneoplastic syndromes.

1- Biological inflammatory syndrome [72]:

Biological inflammatory syndrome is frequent with :

- A significant increase in SV

- Elevated fibrinogen and CRP levels

- Elevated $alpha_2$ globulins

- Inflammatory anemia

- Hyperleukocytosis

2- Immunological abnormalities :

Immunological abnormalities may be associated with the inflammatory syndrome, particularly in cases of myxoma. These abnormalities are :

- An increase in Ig G

- Hyper-complementemia

- Cryoglobulinemia

- The presence of anti-DNA antibodies [73]

- The presence of rheumatoid factor [74].

- IL 6 secretion [75, 76, 77, 74]: this has been demonstrated in the supernatant of cultured myxomatous cells.

Interleukin plays a role in transforming resting B lymphocytes into active, immunoglobulin-secreting B lymphocytes; the autoantibodies produced are responsible for the biological inflammatory syndrome.

Surgical cure of the tumor results in regression of all these signs. Their reappearance should raise fears of tumor recurrence.

3- Other biological abnormalities :

- Polycythemia in permeable foramen ovale with right-to-left shunt

- Thrombocytosis or thrombocytopenia

- Hemolytic anemia

- Hyper-eosinophilia

-Coagulation disorders that can lead to disseminated intravascular coagulation

Non-specific elevation of certain tumor markers (ACE, CA 125, etc.).

VI- Anatomopathological study :

Paraclinical investigations only provide strong presumptive evidence. Diagnostic certainty can only be provided by histological and immunohistochemical examination of the anatomical specimen.

1- Myxomas:

Myxoma is a carcinologically benign tumor. Whereas it was once thought to be of thrombotic origin, it is now accepted that it is a true tumor developed from a pluripotent mesenchymal cell of the endocardium that can differentiate into smooth muscle cells or endothelial cells [9].

Macroscopically, the majority of myxomas present as a well-individualized, rounded or ovoid intracavitary mass, connected to the SIA by an implant base averaging 1 cm^2 wide.

Few myxomas are pedunculated, with a fine pedicle 4 to 8 cm long attached to the AIS. Sessile forms occur much more rarely, and mainly in the ventricles.

The surface may be smooth or papillary. The number of papillae is highly variable, and at most they produce a grape-like appearance. It may also be bumpy, and sometimes the site of thrombotic deposits.

Its consistency is usually firm, despite the visual impression of fragility. However, it can also be soft, gelatinous and friable, leading to embolisms (photo no. 3).

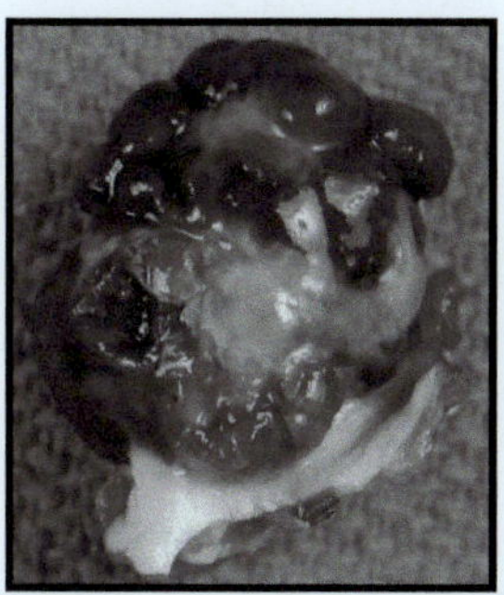

Photo n° 3: Characteristic macroscopic friable, gelatinous and irregular appearance of a cardiac myxoma [22].

Color varies from white-translucent to dark red when there are significant areas of hemorrhage. It is homogeneous in young tumors, but does not remain so in old reworked tumors, where translucent, hemorrhagic and calcified areas alternate.

Weight and size are highly variable: most operated myxomas are larger than 5 cm [78]. The average weight is 35 g (0.75 to 450 g) [38].

The section slice may have a variable appearance: either a gelatinous appearance with myxoid regions and hemorrhagic remodeling, or a hard appearance with collagen fibers. In only 10% of cases are micro-calcifications found [79, 24].

Histological diagnosis of myxomas is based on identification of the myxomatous cells and the myxoid matrix. The latter forms the bulk of the tumor mass. It consists of an amorphous, acidophilic material in which cellular elements are dispersed, often with vascular clefts. Myxomatous cells are round, oval, polygonal or star-shaped. They are isolated or arranged in small clusters, in cords or concentrically around small-calibre vessels (photo no. 4).

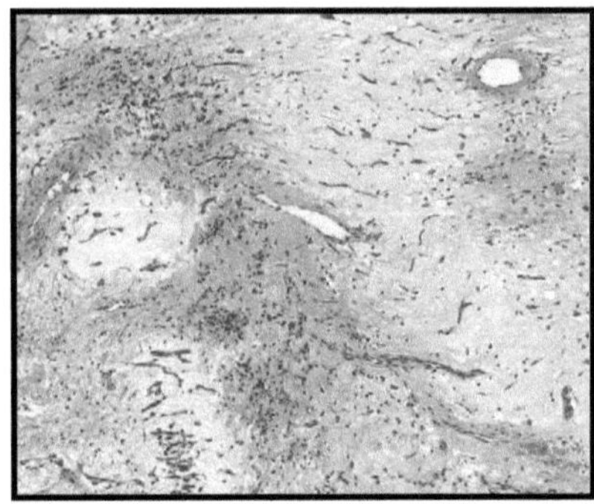

Photo no. 4: Myxomatous cells arranged in cords surrounded by an abundant, collagen-rich myxoid matrix. An infiltrate of mononuclear cells is also present (hematoxylin and eosin, magnification * 200) [22].

Study of the ultrastructure of myxomatous cells reveals that they have the characteristics of primitive mesenchymal cells with an eosinophilic cytoplasm, an oval nucleus with dense chromatin and no visible nucleolus, filaments and tight inter-cellular junctions [80]. Mitoses are rare.

2- Papillary fibroelastomas [81]:

Papillary fibroelastomas are rounded, pedunculated, whitish, mobile formations with a gelatinous surface, sub-centimetric in size.

The histological appearance shows a papillary formation of fine, branched bangs consisting of a central, avascular, peduncular conjunctivo-elastic axis, surrounded by a thin layer of extra-cellular matrix. The matrix is rich in MPS and covered by one or more layers of endothelial cells and smooth muscle cells (photo no. 5).

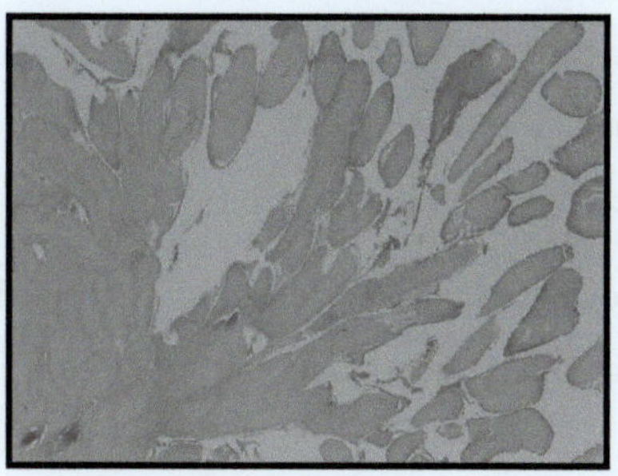

Photo n° 5: Microscopic appearance of papillary fibroelastomas [22].

3- **Inflammatory** pseudotumors **[82]:**

Macroscopically, they are represented by small, homogeneous, pedunculated masses.

Histologically, ITP is a heterogeneous lesion composed of a benign proliferation of inflammatory and mesenchymal cells [9]. This infiltrate is composed essentially of plasma cells, lymphocytes, PNEs, macrophages and myofibroblastic cells with a fibrous stroma (photo no. 6).

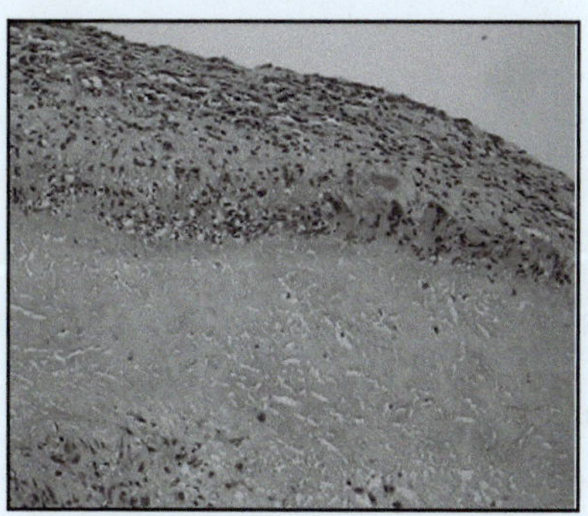

Photo no. 6: Cross-section of mitral valve ITP showing macrophages and inflammatory cells [83].

According to Coffin et al [30], the main histological features are the myxoid, vascular and inflammatory appearance of the matrix; the presence of collagen fibers; and the presence of inflammatory cells.

Kelly et al [84] consider that the absence of cellular atypia, the often pedunculated appearance of the tumor and the good long-term prognosis differentiate ITPs from low-grade sarcomas.

4- Sarcomas:

Angiosarcomas are lobulated, spongy, poorly limited, invasive tumors, brown to violet in color and up to 10 cm in diameter. They contain necrotic and hemorrhagic zones.

Two types of sarcoma have been described:

- In one, the tumor is large, pedunculated, and protrudes into the heart chamber, where it may obstruct it. This type can be completely resected.

- In the other, more common type, there is extensive infiltration of the tumor into the myocardium, epicardium and pericardium. This type can only be partially resected.

Angiosarcomas are characterized by a sinusoidal histological structure. Vascular structures proliferate and are lined by endothelial cells and a rich reticulin network around the vascular lumen [24]. There are also fissures filled with red blood cells, chains and complex papillary formations.

Rhabdomyosarcomas are large, soft, nodular, intramural and/or intracavitary tumours that can exceed 10 cm in diameter. They contain glycogen-, desmin- and myoglobin-rich rhabdomyoblasts with polymorphic nuclei and eosinophilic cytoplasm [20].

Fibrosarcomas are well-circumscribed, firm, whitish-grey masses of variable size. They contain areas of necrosis and hemorrhage [18]. Histologically, the neoplastic tissue consists of long, homogeneous, dense bundles arranged in a chevron pattern. These bundles are made up of elongated cells with oval nuclei, sparse cytoplasm, abundant reticulin and poorly visible boundaries.

Leiomyosarcomas are sessile or pedunculated, with an irregular, sometimes poly-lobed surface. These tumors are soft, with a broad infiltrative base extending over the SIA or SIV, posterior wall and valves. They are yellowish in color, with necrotic-hemorrhagic areas (photo no. 7).

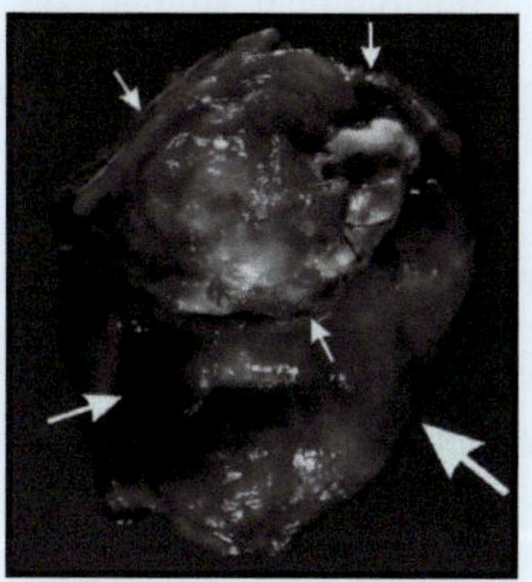

Photo 7: External appearance of cardiac leiomyosarcoma with irregular surface [85].

They are malignant mesenchymal tumors composed of cells with structural or antigenic differentiations from smooth muscle cells. They have a wide spectrum of histological aspects, ranging from low to high degree of atypia.

Cardiac osteosarcomas appear as bulky, sessile masses of firm consistency, 4-6 cm in diameter. They are whitish in color, with central necrotic areas. Histologically, they are extra-cellular osteoid deposits. They are composed of clusters of small spindle-shaped cells with blunt nuclei, frequent areas of necrosis and mitosis, and foci of osteoid deposits surrounded by atypical osteoblastic cells [9].

Liposarcomas appear as small nodules in the OG or OD and rarely the VG, yellowish-white in color and cerebroid in consistency. Histologically, they consist of polymorphous cells arranged in a beach-like pattern within a highly vascularized myxoid stroma. Cells are rounded, variable in size and hyperchromatic in nucleus. Some cells have intra-cytoplasmic vacuoles with lipid-rich contents.

The macroscopic appearance of undifferentiated sarcomas is similar to that of other cardiac sarcomas. Despite histological studies, these cardiac sarcomas remain unclassified because they lack a specific ultrastructure.

Lymphomas are typically multiple, firm and yellowish in color. They form a polypoid mass invading the myocardium and pericardium. The diagnosis of malignant lymphoma can be confirmed by pericardial fluid analysis or pericardial biopsy. Histologically, they are characterized by a high proliferation of B lymphocytes [23].

Fibroids are typically solitary, well circumscribed but not encapsulated, firm, greyish in color with central calcifications (photo no. 8).

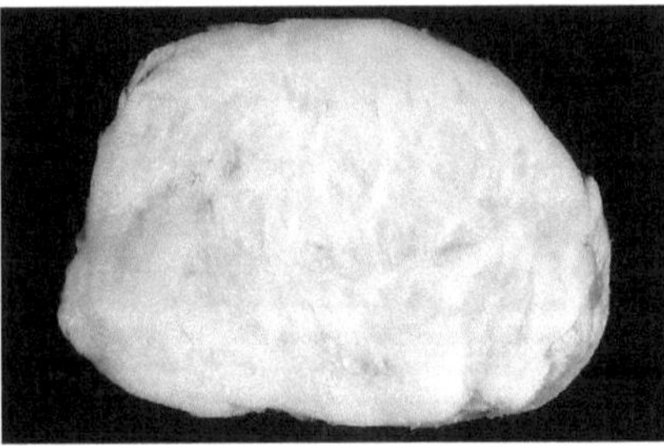

Photo 8: Macroscopic appearance of a ventricular fibroma [86].

Histologically, they constitute a homogeneous proliferation of fibroblast-like cells in a stroma rich in collagen fibers. It is poorly vascularized and contains necrotic-hemorrhagic zones that are often calcified (photo no. 9).

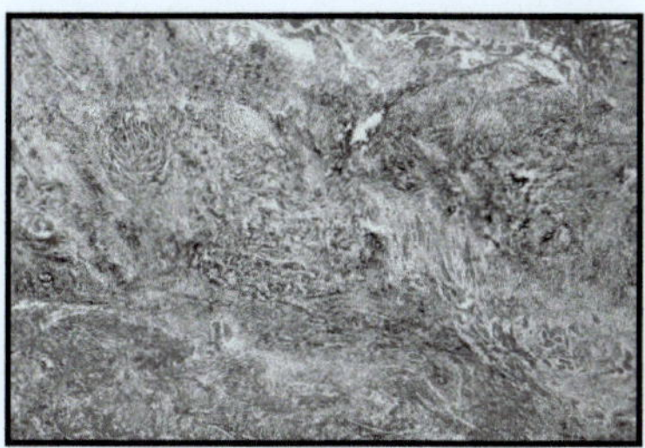

Photo no. 9: Ventricular fibroma (blue) invading myocardial tissue (red) [86].

Cardiac metastases are usually multiple and small. Solitary metastases are rare. The histology of cardiac metastases depends on the histological type of the primary neoplasia.

Photo 10 shows the histological and immunohistochemical appearance of a cardiac metastasis of melanoma [87].

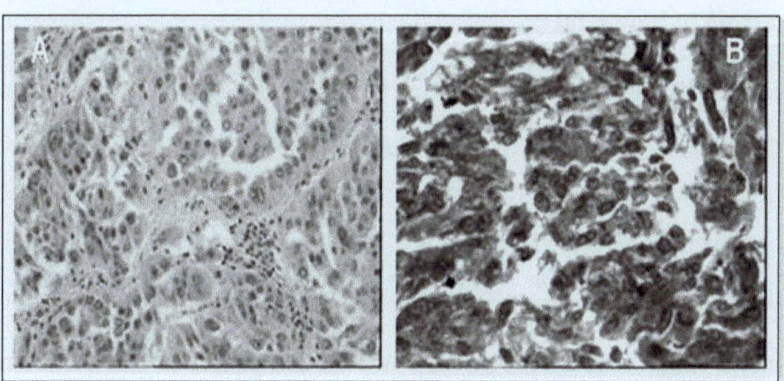

Photo n° 10: Histological examination of a cardiac melanoma [87].

Lipomatous hypertrophy of the AIS leads to an increase in the thickness of the AIS, which protrudes into the OG. It is well-limited, forming a rounded, non-encapsulated mass, most often respecting the fossa ovale. The lesion often measures 2 to 3 cm and can reach up to 15 cm in diameter (photo no. 11).

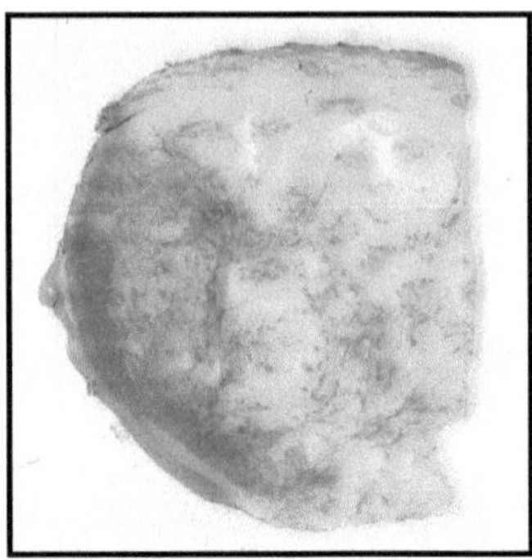

Photo n° 11: Lipomatous hypertrophy of the AIS: large, non-encapsulated mass [88].

Lipomatous hypertrophy of the AIS is characterized by fat accumulation in the AIS in continuity with epicardial fat [13]. It results from hyperplasia of multi-vacuolated adipose cells, with vesicular cytoplasm rich in the mitochondria characteristic of brown fat.

Pericardial mesotheliomas present as bulky nodules in the pericardial cavity, and tend to invade the myocardium and adjacent structures. They have the same histological features as pleural mesotheliomas. They are characterized by the presence of cleft-like formations, bordered by an endothelial and pseudoganglionic lining.

The usual macroscopic presentation of rhabdomyomas is rhabdomyomatosis with multiple nodules, appearing in cross-section as rounded, well-demarcated but non-encapsulated masses. The nodules are located in the ventricular wall, sometimes protruding beneath the epicardium or endocardium.

Microscopic study of the cells reveals that they have the characteristics of striated muscle cells. They are rich in glycogen and lack mitotic activity [24].

Hemangiomas are well-circumscribed, encapsulated masses. They are benign vascular tumors of variable size, which can develop from the epicardium or myocardium, and can also be intra-cavitary (photo no. 12).

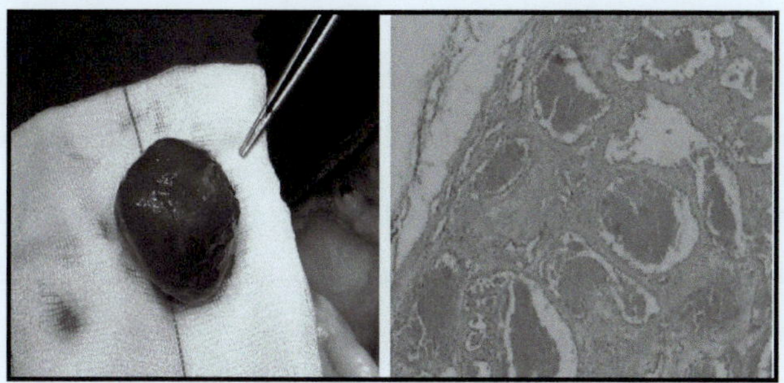

Photo 12: Macroscopic appearance of encapsulated hemorrhage and histological appearance showing proliferation of large vessels with myxoid stroma [89].

VII- Tumor extension [90, 32]:

Malignant cardiac tumors are characterized by rapid growth. At the time of diagnosis, 25% to 30% of primary tumors have metastatic spread.

Secondary localizations are mainly intra-thoracic. The most frequent site is the lung. Next come the mediastinum, pleura, liver, bone, central nervous system, adrenal glands, colon, diaphragm, thyroid, skin, kidneys, pancreas, spleen...

For this reason, extension workup for cardiac sarcomas should include a chest X-ray supplemented by a thoracic CT scan, abdominal ultrasound, bone scan and brain scan.

VIII- Complications :

Primary and secondary cardiac tumors can cause a number of complications:

1- Cardiac rhythm disorders [49, 91]:

Recurrent ventricular arrhythmias are frequently encountered in children with cardiac fibrillation, and can lead to sudden death. These arrhythmias are essentially fibrillation and ventricular tachycardia.

Myocardial infiltration by sarcomas can also trigger supraventricular tachycardia or nodal rhythm.

Complete arrhythmia due to atrial fibrillation is a fairly frequent rhythmic complication of atrial tumors. It is most common in lipomatous hypertrophy of the AIS.

2- Atrioventricular conduction disorders :

Complete atrioventricular block may be the consequence of tumor invasion of the conduction system.

3- Systemic embolisms:

Because of their mobile nature and the hemodynamic constraints to which they are subjected, myxomas are frequently a source of systemic embolisms. Emboli may be formed by thrombotic material detached from the surface of the myxoma, or by a more or less voluminous fringe of the myxoma itself. In rare cases, a whole myxoma may migrate due to rupture of the pedicle.

The trigger for migration appears to be physical activity, exacerbating hemodynamic stress and repeated postural modifications.

The overall frequency of arterial embolism in patients with cardiac myxoma varies from 20 to 60%, with a mean frequency of 45% [92].

The embolic event is often indicative of the tumor. Of the 138 myxomas reported by Mac Allister [40, 41, 42], 36 were complicated by an inaugural embolism and 18 by a secondary embolism. Moreover, embolic events are often recurrent or even multiple [93, 94].

Embolic complications are also common in papillary fibroelastoma, either through tumor fragmentation or detachment of cruoric formations from the tumor surface.

- **Cerebral embolisms:** The cerebral territory is involved in almost half of all cases. Neurological complications will be studied separately.

- **Coronary embolism:** often accompanied by inaugural MI or acute coronary syndrome [95, 41, 96, 97].

- **Embolism in the abdominal aorta:** In this case, the clinical picture is characterized by shock, flaccid paralysis, paresthesia of the lower limbs with lumbar pain and anuria [98].

- **Visceral embolisms:** less frequent than cerebral embolisms.

- **Retinal embolisms:** These can be misleadingly suggestive of Horton's arteritis, given the association of an inflammatory syndrome with ocular signs.

Embolism of the central retinal artery results in unilateral and usually permanent blindness; transient amaurosis is very rare.

4- Pulmonary embolisms:

For tumors located in the right heart, embolization is performed in the lungs. The severity of embolization varies. The embolus may be a tumor fragment or a fibrino-cruciferous thrombus formed within the tumor.

5- Paradoxical embolisms:

Rare cases of paradoxical embolism have been reported [47, 99]. These embolisms were first described by Powers [100] in connection with an OG myxoma through an AIC.

6- Heart failure:

Tumors of the left heart can have an insidious evolution, revealing themselves as left heart failure or even global heart failure.

7- Pulmonary hypertension:

Pulmonary hypertension following multiple embolisms has been described in a few cases [101].

8- Arterial aneurysms:

This is a myxomatous degeneration of the arterial wall in contact with a tumor embolus. The tumor tissue destroys the vascular wall, leaving only tumor cells and a few collagen trabeculae of the adventitia between the lumen and surrounding tissue. These aneurysms then evolve in a completely autonomous fashion, which explains their discovery, and above all their rupture, many years after lumpectomy [102].

These complications can occur in all arterial territories, but are particularly serious when they occur in the brain.

9- Deep vein thrombosis :

Loire [103] reported the possibility of inferior vena cava obstruction leading to Budd Chiari syndrome.

10- Pericardial effusions:

Pericardial effusions can complicate mesothelioma. They are often hemorrhagic, and may progress to recurrent pericarditis, tamponade or chronic pericardial constriction.

11- Neurological complications:

The neurological accident is often the first to occur, and wrongly refers the patient to a neurological center. The main lesion is cerebral embolism, but the anatomo-clinical forms engendered by embolism are multiple and of varying severity.

- **Acute cerebral softening [92]:** This is the most common complication.

Cerebral infarction is due to acute arterial obliteration by a tumor fragment or by fibrino-platelet material developed on the tumor. The ischemic event may be transient, regressive or permanent.

Embolisms are frequently repetitive, with recurrence occurring at great intervals in various cerebral arterial territories, more often in the carotid than in the vertebro-basilar territory, resulting in multiple foci of encephalic ischemia [93].

Multiple repetitive infarctions of this kind can lead to progressive dementia, as in the case of Hutton [94] or Mattle [95]. The latter observation concerns a young child whose dementia syndrome continued to progress after surgical cure of the myxoma.

- **Encephalic aneurysms:** Cases of late-onset aneurysms remote from surgical treatment of myxoma have been reported [92].

Burton [104], Price [105] and Loeper [106] have explained the development of these aneurysms by the destruction of the internal elastic boundary and the media by the tumor tissue of the embolus.

These aneurysms are almost always multiple, distal in location, and vary in size up to 2.5 cm. They are usually fusiform. These lesions are often asymptomatic, but their evolution remains uncertain. A few cases of rupture have been reported [107, 105, 108].

- Intracerebral **metastases:** the arterial wall is breached, allowing tumor cells to pass into the subarachnoid spaces and invade the brain.

12- Myxoma infection:

This is a rare complication. Only a handful of cases have been published in the literature [14].

This is a surgical emergency to prevent the occurrence of a septic embolus, which would be catastrophic for the brain [79].

13- Sudden death:

Tumors of the heart, whatever their histological type, may be discovered at autopsy after sudden death. This is related to a massive embolic coronary or pulmonary accident, acute obstruction of a valvular orifice or a severe rhythm disorder.

IX- Differential diagnosis :

1- Cardiac hydatid cysts:

The ultrasonographic characteristics of hydatid cysts with a liquid content distinguish them from tumors with a solid echostructure.

2- Infective endocarditis :

Valvular tumors can be confused with vegetations of infective endocarditis. Differentiation is made by TEE.

3- Thrombi:

Although echocardiography remains the essential test for the diagnosis of intracavitary thrombi, a number of false positives have been reported in the literature. In these situations, MRI can help in the diagnosis: a thrombus appears hyper-signal on T1- and T2-weighted images when fresh, and hypo-signal when organized.

Progression under anti-coagulant treatment will confirm the diagnosis.

Hiroaki Konichi et al [109] described a case of organized thrombus of the tricuspid valve mistaken for a valvular tumour. The diagnosis of thrombus was established by histological examination of the surgical specimen.

4- Lambl's outgrowths [110]:

There is a histological similarity between papillary fibroelastomas and Lambl's excrescences. The distinction between these two entities is based on their location and size.

Lambl's excrescences are located on the Arantius nodule, the free edge or confrontation zone of sigmoid valves, and on the atrial side of the confrontation zone of atrioventricular valves. In contrast, fibroelastomas are often found on the ventricular side of sigmoid valves and on the atrial side of atrioventricular valves, outside the confrontation zones and free edge, and more rarely on the cords and on the atrial and ventricular endocardium.

Fibroelastomas are also larger than Lambl's excrescences, averaging 1 cm and up to 5 cm in size.

5- Connectivites:

The presence of cutaneous manifestations and immunological disturbances can lead to a variety of pictures more or less suggestive of collagenosis. These are known as pseudo-lupus syndrome, rheumatoid arthritis or polymyositis. Other conditions, such as rheumatic fever, periarteritis nodosa and Horton's disease in elderly patients with retinal embolism, may also be considered.

But wrong diagnoses must be revised after a few weeks or months of ineffective treatment.

Garnier [92], in 8 cases of OG myxomas with neurological manifestations, noted a pseudo-lupus syndrome which led to the diagnosis being misinterpreted for several months.

X- Processing :

1- Surgical treatment :

The excision of cardiac tumors is a relatively recent technique, since in 1954 the first left atrial myxoma was successfully removed by Crafoord under CEC [5].

1- 1- Goals :

- **Tumor resection:** Resection of the tumor removes the mechanical obstacle to blood flow and prevents embolic complications. Resection must be performed en bloc to avoid embolization of tumor fragments in the pulmonary arterial circulation.

Tumor manipulation must also be kept to a minimum, due to the risk of fragmentation and tumor embolization.

- **Prevention of recurrence:** To prevent tumor recurrence, most authors recommend wide excision, not only of the tumor mass but also of the surrounding area of healthy myocardial and endocardial tissue.
- **Exploration of the four cardiac cavities:** Macroscopic exploration of the cardiac cavities is a procedure recommended by several authors, because sometimes, during the initial radiological work-up, a second or more tumours located in another cavity may have gone undetected [111].
- **Checking valve function:** intra-cavity tumors can interfere with valve function, so it's essential to check valve function and, if necessary, perform an annuloplasty or valve replacement.

1- 2- Indications :

- **General indications:** As soon as a cardiac tumor is diagnosed, intervention is essential, as the spontaneous evolution, irrespective of the histological nature, can be sudden death.

In such cases, the ideal time between diagnosis and surgery should be no more than a few days, whatever the tumour location. Early intervention often results in a better quality of life. It also means better local tumor control, and potentially better survival in the case of malignant tumors.

The presence of metastases at the time of diagnosis is not considered a contraindication to surgical excision of malignant tumors by the majority of authors.

- Special cases :

Papillary fibroelastomas: The treatment of papillary fibroelastomas is the subject of controversy. Some suggest systematic surgical resection, while others recommend periodic surveillance with anti-coagulation for asymptomatic patients with immobile tumors [112].

Lipomas: Only the existence of a severe obstructive syndrome or pericardial compression revealed by echocardiography or MRI justifies radical surgical treatment.

Lipomatous hypertrophy of the IAT: The surgical indications for lipomatous hypertrophy of the IAT are obstruction of the superior vena cava and the presence of cardiac rhythm disorders.

Rhabdomyomas and fibroids [113]: Rhabdomyomas may regress spontaneously, or even involve completely, justifying simple regular ultrasound monitoring in the absence of symptoms.

Opinions differ on the treatment of asymptomatic fibroids: the risk of sudden arrhythmic death has led some teams to retain the surgical indication, while others prefer close clinical and ultrasound monitoring until clinical symptoms appear.

On the other hand, the prognosis for severe symptomatic forms (obstructive syndrome, severe rhythm disorders) is poor, leading to the suggestion of rapid surgical treatment of cardiac fibromas and rhabdomyomas.

Cardiac metastases: In most cases of cardiac metastases, the invasion is diffuse and makes excision impossible [114]. In such cases, palliative partial resection may be proposed.

1- 3- Approach :

- **Sternotomy:** The classic approach currently used by most surgeons is the median sternotomy. It enables rapid and easy installation of the CEC, and tumor removal under optimum conditions, by allowing access to all four cavities.
- **Mini-sternotomy:** Superior mini-sternotomy was used by Indra et al [80] for the resection of two left atrial myxomas.
- **Thoracotomy:** Right and left antero-lateral thoracic approaches are now being used less and less.

Botta et al described a case of intrapericardial lipoma successfully excised through a right anterolateral thoracotomy [115].

- **Video surgery:** The concept of minimally invasive surgery with laparoscopy has recently been introduced to treat cardiac lesions, including tumor resection surgery. This method is safe, effective and well tolerated. It has lower morbidity and mortality than conventional surgery.

It is performed through a right paraspinal mini-incision and under femorofemoral bypass. Arterial and venous cannula positioning is guided by intraoperative TEE [116].

Jennifer F et al [117] used video-assisted surgery through a 4 cm right mini-thoracotomy in the resection of a huge subepicardial lipoma of the OD compressing both vena cava.

1- 4- Extracorporeal circulation :

Surgical treatment is always performed under CEC, the only way to obtain a bloodless surgical field and an immobile heart, essential conditions for achieving the objectives of radical surgical treatment.

Aortic cannulation is performed below the start of the brachiocephalic arterial trunk. Cannulation of the superior and inferior vena cava must be performed with great care, as it may result in mobilization of a tumor fragment.

Remote cannulation of the femoral vein, superior vena cava, internal jugular vein or innominate venous trunk is sometimes justified. In the case of atrial localization, vena cava is essential to completely isolate the heart from the bloodstream.

The heart is stopped either by fibrillation, after placement of epicardial electrodes without aortic clamping, or by total cardiac arrest through hypothermia and injection of cold cardioplegia at the root of the aorta at the moment of aortic clamping. This has now become the technique of choice. The aspiration of blood from the operating field during tumour resection and its reinjection into the pump is controversial, given the risk of intraoperative dissemination of tumour cells [118].

1- 5- Tumor exposure routes :

The best surgical approach should :

- Enable minimal tumor manipulation
- Provide adequate exposure to ensure complete tumor resection
- Allows inspection of all four chambers of the heart
- Minimize the risk of recurrence

Several routes have been proposed for approaching and extracting the tumor:

- **Right auriculotomy (photo no. 13):** It is ideally suited to tumors of the DO and tricuspid valve.

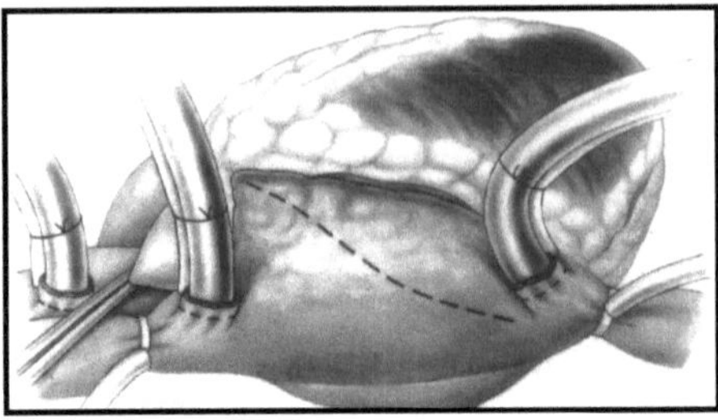

Photo no. 13: Oblique right auriculotomy [119].

- **Left auriculotomy**: Left auriculotomy is used to locate the insertion of a tumor in the OG or mitral valve.

However, it has a number of drawbacks [120, 35]:

- When the OG is only slightly dilated, this approach allows only a limited incision and difficult access to the cavity, and may hinder the removal of a large tumor.

- It does not allow good exposure of the AIS, and can therefore make excision of the base of myxoma implantation difficult.

- It makes it difficult to close any septal breach.

- It prevents proper verification of the right side of the AIS, which may be invaded by the myxoma.

- It requires excessive manipulation of the left atrial tumour and, if large, may escape complete excision.

- **The bi-auricular route:** First used by Cooley in 1973 [7], it is currently adopted by several teams [120, 121, 122, 123]. Two methods are possible:

- Either separate opening of the two earpieces (photo no. 14)

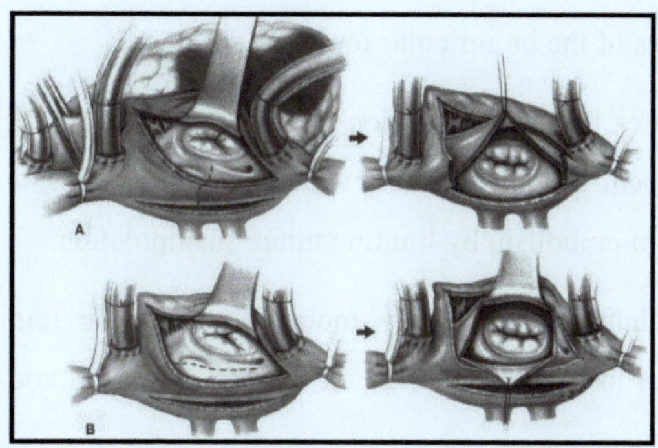

Photo no. 14: Bi-atrial tract with septal incision [119].

A: Parallel right and left vertical auriculotomies with transverse septal incision perpendicular to the auriculotomies passing through the fossa ovale.

B: parallel right and left vertical auriculotomies with vertical septal incision parallel to the auriculotomies.

- Either both auricles and the septum are opened by the same incision (photo no. 15).

The incision is made horizontally along the axis of the superior pulmonary veins.

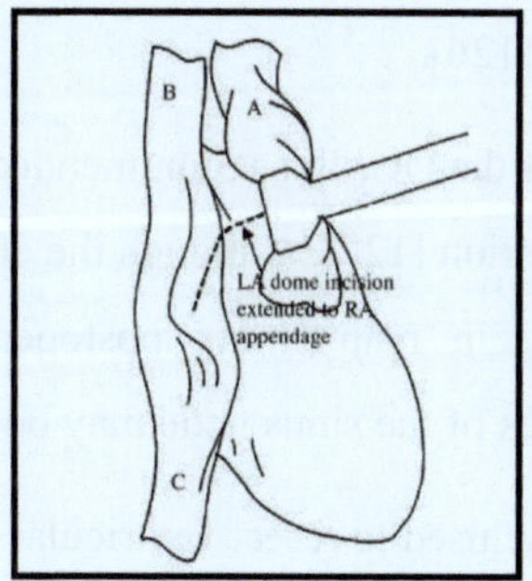

Photo n° 15: Schematic representation of the bi-auricular approach through a single incision [124].

The advantages of the bi-auricular route are :

- It facilitates the externalization of large tumors and excessively friable tumors, as the opening is always very wide, which, as Marvasti [46] points out, reduces the risk of embolism by limiting tumor manipulation.

- This technique avoids any mobilization of the tumor, and allows exploration of all the heart's cavities, as well as the mitral and tricuspid valve apparatus.

- This approach is indicated in cases of bi-atrial tumor localization.

The major disadvantage of this approach is that it can be responsible for a high rate of arrhythmias and early and late post-operative conduction disorders [125]. This is linked to surgical lesions of the conduction pathways.

- **The supra-septal approach:** The DO is incised longitudinally, at a distance from the inter-auriculoventricular groove. The inter-atrial septum is opened vertically to the inferior border of the fossa ovale, with a 2 cm extension of this incision to the superior border of the latter. The right auriculotomy is then extended superiorly between the right atrium and the inter-auriculoventricular groove to join the upper end of the septal incision. When these two incisions meet, the roof of the OG is opened [126].

It offers excellent exposure of the OG. It is recommended when the OG is small, and in the event of re-intervention [127]. Although the efficacy of this technique has been proven, its safety in maintaining postoperative sinus rhythm is controversial, since the arteries of the sinus node may be damaged [128, 129].

- **Transverse aortotomy:** used to resect ventricular tumors.

1- 6- Tumor extraction:

- **Myxomas:** The problems posed by the extraction of myxomatous tumors are :

- Tumor friability: there is a risk of fragmentation and migration of tumor fragments during intra-operative manipulations, resulting in myxomatous embolism.

- Extent of resection: two attitudes have been adopted by authors:

- Maximumist approach: the majority of authors [125, 7] recommend wide excision, not only of the base of myxoma implantation, but also of the surrounding area of healthy myocardial tissue; and systematic exploration of all 4 cavities to minimize the risk of recurrence.

- Conservative approach: involves resecting the tumor and a small portion of the surrounding endocardium [130].

Approach: the extent of the resection also dictates the approach. Thus, the right atrial approach with septal incision and bi-atrial approaches enable extensive excisions [7]. Left auriculotomy allows complete excision of small OG myxomas or large myxomas after fragmentation and aspiration of the fragments [131].

For left atrial myxomas, Bortolotti [125] distinguished two cases:

- The implant base is located at the level of the fossa ovale: in this case, the SIA is removed over a wide area and through its entire thickness, creating an AIC; and the resulting septal defect is repaired according to its size by simple suture; or by a patch.

- In this case, only the endocardium surrounding the tumor and part of the underlying myocardium are excised. The area involved is therefore smaller than in the first case, and a simple suture repair may suffice.

- **Papillary fibroelastomas:** In the majority of cases, complete surgical resection of the mass with preservation of the native valve is possible and sufficient. Wider resection requiring valve replacement may also be necessary [48].

- **Inflammatory pseudotumors:** resection surgery for ITPs follows the same rules as for myxomas.

- **Rhabdomyomas and fibroids**: Complete resection of congenital tumours, justified by the risk of arrhythmias and sudden death, is not always possible. In such cases, partial resection is indicated [132].

- **Malignant tumors:** The removal of malignant tumors must comply with the following rules:

- Ventricular massage and dislocation should be avoided prior to aortic clamping, due to the friability of tumors and the risk of pulmonary embolism.

- Cannulas must be inserted with care.

- There needs to be wide access to both atria, enabling both sides of the SIA and the mitral and tricuspid valve apparatus to be checked.

Surgical resection may or may not be complete, depending on the location and size of the tumour and its extension into the myocardium. In patients whose tumor is limited to the free wall of the atrium, the atrial septum or the valve, complete resection may be envisaged. The difficulty of exposing the posterior portion of the heart is the major challenge in resecting posterior tumors. Complete heart detachment followed by tumour resection and heart reimplantation is used by some teams [133, 134, 85, 135].

The total resectability rate reported in the largest series of cardiac sarcomas varies from 33 to 75% [136].

1- 7- Associated valve procedures:

Traumatic valve lesions may be caused by large tumours embedded in the mitral or tricuspid orifice [122]. In such cases, progressive deterioration of the valve condition rarely necessitates valve replacement.

Conservative surgery is preferred to valve replacement [125, 47]. Saint John Sutton [38] reported only one replacement out of 40 myxoma procedures.

1- 8- Heart transplantation [137] :

It has recently been introduced as a palliative treatment for malignant tumors of the heart. A history of cancer is classically considered an absolute contraindication to heart transplantation.

Heart transplantation is only proposed in cases of local recurrence after surgical excision, or for unresectable, non-metastatic tumors. It is performed after neoadjuvant chemotherapy.

Because of the limited number of published cases, the lack of experience with this technique, the long waiting times to obtain a compatible graft, and the deleterious effects of immunosuppressive treatment in these patients, heart transplantation is not currently a therapeutic standard, but a research avenue that requires further investigation.

1- 9- Tumor resection with cardiac auto-transplantation [133, 85]:

Complete resection of deep, posterior tumors with a heart in place can be difficult or impossible to achieve, and may cause early post-operative recurrence. For this reason, externalization of the heart outside the mediastinal cavity can solve the problem of exposure. This is achieved by sectioning both vena cava and the great vessels, followed by ex-vivo tumor resection, reconstruction of the cavities with an autologous or bovine pericardial patch, and reimplantation of the heart.

It has been used by several teams as an alternative to heart transplantation for the treatment of unresectable invasive tumors.

1-10- The end of the intervention :

This is the stage when the integrity of the four heart chambers is verified. Careful washing of the cavities with saline solution is essential to avoid leaving any tumour debris that could embolize in the immediate post-operative period or cause early recurrence.

After suturing the auriculotomies, purging the left cavities, declamping, warming up, and after the heart's rhythm has returned (spontaneously or by defibrillation), bypass surgery is gradually stopped, if the heart's hemodynamic state allows. Finally, the surgeon closes the chest, after pericardial and mediastinal drainage.

2- Radiotherapy:

Radiotherapy is considered a complementary therapy to surgery for malignant tumors. Radiation energy and technique are adapted on a case-by-case basis.

2- 1- Sarcomas :

Irradiation is often performed using a linear gas pedal. Cobalt has only been used by a few authors [138].

The dose to be delivered is 50 gys. An additional dose of 10 gys is recommended in the event of macroscopic residue, without exceeding the tolerance of sensory neighboring structures (lungs, spinal chains) [139]. The dose per fraction is 1.8 to 2 gys, with one fraction per day and 5 fractions per week [140].

There is no standard definition of the volume to be irradiated. The entire operating bed, including the drain path and orifices, must be involved, with a large safety margin [141].

Radiotherapy in cardiac sarcomas is only conceivable as an adjunctive treatment after surgical excision, or as a palliative treatment if the tumour is unresectable [140, 142]. It should be performed as close as possible to surgical excision, with a desirable delay of less than 5 weeks. Neoadjuvant radiotherapy aimed at reducing the tumour mass preoperatively has no place because of the extent of the volume to be irradiated.

The choice of radiotherapy is limited by the frequency and severity of its acute complications such as pericarditis, fever and pain; and its chronic complications of constrictive pericarditis and coronary artery stenosis [143].

2- 2- **Inflammatory** pseudotumors :

Radiotherapy has been used by some teams for the treatment of ITPs for which complete excision was impossible, although its beneficial effect in this type of tumor has not been proven [144].

2- 2- Mesotheliomas and lymphomas :

Radiotherapy has not proved effective in the treatment of mesothelioma and cardiac lymphoma.

3- Chemotherapy [140, 145]:

3- 1- Sarcomas:

Chemotherapy is increasingly used as an adjunctive treatment after complete or partial surgical resection of cardiac sarcomas with or without metastases. Neo-adjuvant chemotherapy is justified when local extension does not allow complete resection, which becomes possible after reduction of tumour size by chemotherapy.

A review of the literature reveals some isolated successes with the combination of surgery and chemotherapy, but there is no real consensus on the best therapeutic strategy [146, 147, 148]. The only consensus to date concerns surgery. Indeed, the need for as complete a resection as possible as the first therapeutic gesture is the convention of authors, especially with the progress in cardiac surgery.

The role of complementary treatment with chemotherapy and/or radiotherapy and their respective indications in the treatment of sarcomas remains to be established. Some authors propose triple therapy (surgery + chemotherapy + radiotherapy); others reject it on the grounds that anthracyclines increase the cardiac toxicity of radiotherapy [146]. Several chemotherapy protocols such as CYVADIC (cyclophosphamide, vincristine, adriamycin, imidazole, carboxamide) have been used with variable results. A large meta-analysis [149] of the use of doxorubicin in cardiac sarcoma concluded that it significantly reduced local recurrence and metastases, and improved survival.

3- 2- Lymphomas :

Several randomized trials [10, 150] have demonstrated the benefits of anthracycline-based chemotherapy followed by radiotherapy in the treatment of lymphomas. Prolonged complete remissions have been described after combined chemotherapy and radiotherapy.

3-3- Pericardial mesotheliomas :

Chemotherapy plays a palliative role in the treatment of pericardial mesotheliomas.

4- Gene therapy :

Several clinical studies have shown that the new tyrosine kinase inhibitors have beneficial effects in slowing the progression of cardiac sarcomatous disease [151, 150].

Nakagawa et al [150] recommend the use of anti-CD 20 monoclonal antibodies (rituximab) for non-Hodgkin's B lymphomas expressing the CD 20 molecule. This is an effective new therapy for this type of lymphoma.

Induction of apoptosis in cancer cells is another new therapeutic alternative. However, given the effect of apoptosis on normal myocardial cells inducing heart failure, this approach merits clinical trials before being applied [151].

5- Anti-coagulation :

Medical treatment with long-term anti-coagulation or anti-aggregation is discussed according to tumour location and whether or not the patient's general condition contraindicates surgery [22].

6- Anti-arrhythmics :

Anti-arrhythmics are indicated in non-operable fibroids complicated by recurrent ventricular rhythm disorders [91].

XI- Prognosis and survival :

1- Natural evolution:

- Benign tumors :

The majority of benign tumors, because of their numerous complications, present a significant risk to the patient's life expectancy. Systematic surgical cure should therefore be undertaken even in the case of a clinically silent tumour (except for the histological types mentioned above), to avoid any complication that would necessitate an emergency procedure and worsen an initially excellent prognosis.

The spontaneous prognosis of ITP is often favorable. However, some cases of transformation into sarcomas and sudden death have been described [152]. Spontaneous regression of the tumour has also been described [153, 154].

- Malignant tumors :

The prognosis for patients with malignant tumors is poor. Spontaneous evolution rapidly leads to locoregional and distant invasion, culminating in death.

The average survival of sarcoma patients is no more than one year after the onset of symptoms [136, 11].

2- Therapeutic results :

- Benign tumors :

Early post-operative results are excellent, provided that all the intra-operative precautions already mentioned are observed. The series published in the literature report a low rate of early post-operative mortality [120, 125]. The main causes of death are ventricular rhythm disorders, systemic embolic events, and low flow in the event of preoperative myocardial dysfunction [155].

Early post-operative complications are generally limited to conduction disorders or rhythm disturbances, which usually resolve within a few days, aided by the bi-atrial approach and wide incisions.

Tschirkov [130] asserted that the risk of postoperative arrhythmia is directly proportional to the size of the portion of endocardium removed with the tumor. This author recommended that this removal should be kept to a minimum.

Late mortality rates for myxoma vary in the literature from 0 to 25% [125, 111]. However, it seems that the majority of late deaths are not attributable to the operation, but to any other cause not directly related to the myxoma. However, a few cases of late neurological events revealing latent cerebral aneurysms have been reported [156].

Recurrence is rare. Most series report little or no recurrence [157, 123]. Recurrence can occur in several ways: as a single tumor or multiple tumors, in the same cavity as the initial tumor or in another cavity.

The etiologies of recurrences are :

- Incomplete excision of the initial tumor

- Migration of tumor fragments during surgery

- The initial presence of another tumour location that has gone unnoticed

- Myxoma runs in families

An assessment of the overall recurrence rate was given by Castelli [157] in a literature review of 526 myxomas. This rate was estimated at 4.7%, with significant variations between subgroups.

The rate of spontaneous local recurrence of ITP varies from 15% to 37%. It is highest in the first year after surgery [158]. A subgroup of patients at high risk of recurrence has been identified: familial forms, forms associated with Carney complex syndrome, and multiple forms. The occurrence of pre-operative neurological complications clouds the tumor's prognosis. In a review of the literature, Roeltgen [159] reported a morbidity rate of 49%, which contrasts with the excellent prognosis of operated myxomas uncomplicated by brain lesions.

- **Malignant tumors :**

The early post-operative mortality rate was estimated at 12.5% in the series by Donsbeck [160] and Burke [136], involving 24 and 40 patients respectively operated on for cardiac sarcomas.

Tumor resection surgery followed by adjuvant chemotherapy improves patient survival [18, 151]. The frequency of local invasion and distant metastases at the time of diagnosis of rhabdomyosarcomas and their poor response to radiotherapy and chemotherapy limit the survival of patients after surgery to less than 12 months [136, 23].

2- Prognostic elements:

- **Quality of surgical excision:** The factor consistently and significantly found to be the quality of surgical excision during initial treatment [161]. Thus, complete tumour resection seems to increase survival [9].

- Tumour location: Left-sided cavities appear to be associated with longer survival. This is probably due to their earlier diagnosis, compared with right-sided cardiac localizations which are often discovered late, making their complete resection more difficult [136, 9].

- Histological grade: directly correlates with survival rate.

In Donsbeck's series [160], the average survival time was longer in patients with low-grade tumors than in those with high-grade tumors (16.7 months versus 7).

- **Histological type:** Chances of survival are excellent for myxomas, average for benign tumors other than myxomas, and poor for malignant neoplasia.

In the majority of series reported in the literature, the histological type of sarcoma does not appear to correlate statistically with survival [9, 160]. However, in a series of 15 cardiac sarcomas reported by Lombart [147], survival was significantly longer in patients without angiosarcoma (18 months versus 7, p= 0.04).

- **Adjuvant treatment**: Post-operative adjuvant treatment with chemotherapy and/or radiotherapy sometimes seems to be associated with a more favorable outcome [136, 160].

In Burke's series [136], mean survival was longer in patients who received additional treatment after surgical resection (19 months vs. 7, p= 0.03).

XII- Conclusion :

Primary cardiopericardial tumors are rare. Their incidence is estimated at around 0.02%. Three-quarters are benign. Myxoma of the OG is the most frequent tumor, followed by lipoma and fibroelastoma.

ITP is an extremely rare benign lesion of unknown etiology.

Primary malignant tumors are also rare, and are represented in 95% of cases by sarcomas. Cardiac metastases are much more frequent, with an incidence 20 to 40 times higher than that of primary tumors. Melanoma and bronchopulmonary cancers have the highest incidence of heart metastases.

The clinical presentation of cardiac tumors is polymorphous and unspecific. It depends more on the location of the tumor and its relationship to conduction tissue and valves than on its size and histological type. Symptoms may include dyspnea, chest pain, malaise, syncope and signs of heart failure.

Certain histological types of tumor are associated with general signs. Tumors with endo-cavitary and valvular development may be responsible for embolism into the coronary, cerebral, renal, pulmonary or peripheral circulation, leading to ischemic accidents.

Pericardial tumors can cause pericardial effusion, tamponade or constrictive pericarditis.

Nearly 12% of primary cardiac tumors are asymptomatic, and the diagnosis is made during an echocardiogram performed for another reason, or at autopsy.

The main advantage of these polymorphous signs is that they prompt a request for a cardiac ultrasound scan, which will more often than not establish the diagnosis. In fact, TTE and TEE are the key diagnostic tests, sufficient to refer the patient to the surgeon.

Ultrasound can also be used to search for valvular or pericardial invasion, assess left ventricular function and guide biopsy in unresectable tumors requiring chemotherapy and/or radiotherapy. However, this technique can be undermined by false positives, false negatives and limited and insufficient analysis of mediastinal tumor extension.

In atypical forms, MRI and, to a lesser extent, CT scans are useful. These methods can be used to confirm the diagnosis by eliminating false positives, and to pinpoint the location and extent of the disease.

CT provides the necessary information on invasion of adjacent structures, the presence of pleural effusion, mediastinal adenopathy and pulmonary metastases. It can also be used to study large vessels. In some cases, MRI can also be used to characterize tissue histology and look for signs of malignancy. It can also be used for post-treatment follow-up of malignant lesions.

The diagnostic value of biology lies in the search for a non-specific biological inflammatory syndrome. Immunological abnormalities can also be found in myxoma patients. IL 6 levels are also used for post-operative monitoring of certain tumors. Elevated plasma levels indicate tumor recurrence.

Anatomopathological study is the key to diagnosing cardiac tumors. Macroscopic appearance varies according to the histological type of tumor.

Myxoma usually presents as a well-individualized intracavitary mass of firm consistency and variable size, connected to the SIA by a broad base of implantation.

Papillary fibroelastoma (PTI) is a rounded, pedunculated, mobile, sub-centimetric formation located on the valvular endocardium. ITP presents as a homogeneous, well-limited mass.

Malignant tumors are poorly limited, invasive, usually multiple, and contain necrotic-hemorrhagic zones.

Pericardial tumors, which are often metastases, present as large nodules. They tend to invade the myocardium and adjacent structures, leading to pericardial effusion.

Histologically, primary and secondary malignant tumors are characterized by frequent cellular atypia and mitosis. The difficulties involved in identifying each type of tumor, as well as the differential diagnosis with other non-tumoral cardiac formations such as thrombi, vegetations and Lambl outgrowths, have only been resolved by the development of electron microscopy, immunohistochemistry and molecular biology techniques.

Immunohistochemical studies identify proteins and receptors expressed on the cell surface to confirm the diagnosis and differentiate histological types. Cytogenetic studies are used to identify links between certain tumors and chromosomal aberrations or gene mutations.

Therapeutic management requires collaboration between the cardiologist, cardiac surgeon and anesthetist.

For malignant tumors, collaboration with the oncologist and radiotherapist is often necessary. The aim of surgical excision is to remove the mechanical obstacle to blood flow and prevent embolic and rhythmic complications, as well as tumor recurrence.

Intraoperative macroscopic exploration of the heart's cavities and verification of valve function are essential.

The most commonly used approach today is the median sternotomy. It allows rapid installation of the CEC and easy access to all cardiac cavities. The ideal route for exposure of the tumor varies according to its location and size. It should allow minimal manipulation of the tumor, inspection of all four heart chambers, and adequate exposure.

The principle of surgery is to ensure complete removal of the tumor with its pedicle and base of implantation, with reconstruction of any valve defect or heart wall.

Heart transplantation after neoadjuvant chemo-radiotherapy is a therapeutic alternative for patients with neoplasia of significant local extension and no distant metastases. However, given the limited number of donors and the morbidity associated with immunosuppression, it is the treatment of last resort.

Chemotherapy is an essential element in the treatment of malignant tumors. It is increasingly used as a complementary treatment after complete or partial surgical resection. However, due to the extreme rarity of malignant tumors, no precise therapeutic protocol has yet been adopted.

Radiotherapy represents the third stage in the treatment of malignant tumors of the heart. In the treatment of cardiac sarcomas, it is only conceivable as a complementary treatment after surgical excision, or as a palliative treatment if the tumor is unresectable.

For benign tumors, radiotherapy is only used for ITPs where complete excision is impossible, although its beneficial effect in this type of tumor has not been proven.

The short- and long-term prognosis after surgery for benign tumors is excellent. Local recurrence is rare. It is often due to incomplete resection. The prognosis for malignant tumors remains poor, despite complete resection and adjuvant treatment.

Regular post-operative follow-up using non-invasive methods is recommended for early detection of recurrence.

Bibliography :

1. International Agency for Research on Cancer. WHO Classification of Tumours of the Lung, Pleura, Thymus and Heart 4th edn (World Health Organization, 2015).

2. Mahaim I. Tumors and polyps of the heart.

Ed. Masson, Paris, 1945.

3. Silverman N.A. Primary cardiac tumors.

Ann. Surg, 1980, 191 (2): 127-38.

4. Norlindh T, Lilja B, Nyman U, Hellekant C.

Left atrial myxoma demonstrated with CT.

Amer J Roentgenol 1981; 1: 153-4.

5. Fisher M, Cherrier F.

Heart myxomas.

Med interne 1980; 15: 277- 83.

6. Isner J, Falcone M, Virmani R, Roberts W.

Cardiac sarcoma causing "ASH" and simulating coronary heart disease.

Amer J Med 1979; 6: 1025-30.

7. Cooley DA.

Surgical treatment of cardiac neoplasms: 32 year experience.

Thorac Cardiovasc Surg 1990; 38: 176-82.

8. Mervin B, Todd M, Edward J.

Cardial myxomas: a clinical diagnosis challenge.

Amer J Surg 1979; 138: 68-76.

9. Burke A, Virmani R.

Tumors of the heart and great vessels.

Atlas of tumor pathology. Third series, fascicle 16. Washington, D.C: Armed Forces Institute of Pathology, 1996; 16: 231.

10. Chomette G, Auriol M, Cabrol C, Tranbaloc P.

Primary malignant tumors of the heart. Anatomo-clinical study of 12 cases.

Ann Med Interne (Paris) 1985; 136: 301-5.

11. Murphy MC, Sweeney MS, Putnam JB, Jr, Walker WE, Frazier OH, Ott DA et al.

Surgical treatment of cardiac tumors: a 25-year experience.

Ann Thorac Surg 1990; 49: 612-7.

12. Carney JA.

Psammomatous melanotic schwanoma. A distinctive, heritable tumor with special associations, including cardiac myxoma and the Cushing syndrome.

Am J Surg Pathol 1990; 14: 206-22.

13. Gaerte SC, Meyer CA, Winer-Muram HT, et al.

Fat-containing lesions of the chest.

Radiographics 2002; 22 (suppl): S 61-78.

14. Furber A, Prunier F, Laporte J et al.

Cardio pericardial tumors. EMC (Paris).

Cardiologie Angeiologie 11-28 A 10, 1999; 10P.

15. Kipfer B, Englberger L, Stauffer E, Carrel T.

Rare presentation of cardiac hemangiomas.

Ann Thorac Surg 2000; 70: 977-9.

16. Abraham K.P, Reddy V, Gattuso P.

Neoplasms metastatic to the heart: review of 3314 consecutive autopsies.

Am J Cardiovasc Pathol 1990; 3: 195-8.

17. Vantrigt P, Sabiston J.R.

Tumors of the heart.

Surgery of the chest, Philadelphia: W.B. Saunders 1995 pp 2069-89.

18. Lam KY, Dickens P, Chan AC.

Tumors of the heart: a 20-year experience with a review of 12,485 consecutive autopsies.

19. Shapiro LM.

Cardiac tumours: diagnosis and management.

Heart 2001; 85: 218-22.

20. Burke A, Virmani R.

Tumors and tumour-like conditions of the heart. In: Silver MD, Gotleib AG, Schoen FJ (eds). Cardiovascular pathology.

New York: Churchill Livingstone, 2001: 583-605.

21. Saad RS, Galvis CO, Bshara W, et al.

Pulmonary valve papillary fibroelastoma: a case report and review of the literature.

Arch Pathol Lab Med 2001; 125: 933-4.

22. Butany J, Nair V, Naseemuddin A, Nair G, Catton C, Yau T.

Cardiac tumours: diagnosis and management.

Lancet Oncology 2005; 6: 219-28.

23. Miralles A, Bracamonte L, Soncul H, Diaz del Castillo R, Akhtar R, Bors V, et al.

Cardiac tumors: clinical experience and surgical results in 74 patients.

Ann Thorac Surg 1991; 52: 886-95.

24. Sarjeant JM, Butany J, Cusimano RJ.

Cancer of the heart: epidemiology and management of primary neoplasms and metastases.

Am J Cardiovasc Drugs 2003; 3: 407-21.

25. Markel ML, Waller BF, Armstrong WF.

Cardiac myxoma: a review.

Medicine 1987; 66: 114-25.

26. Dong Hi AY, Williams CR.

Sex distribution in cardiac myxomas.

Am J Cardiol 2002; 90: 563-5.

27. Goswami KC, Shrivastava S, Bahl VK, Saxena A, Manchauda SC, Wasir HS.

Cardiac myxomas: clinical and echographic profile.

Int J Cardiol 1998; 63: 251-9.

28. Kasis A, Chukwuemeka AO, Vecht JA, Ibrahim MF, Young CP.

An unusual cause of ventricular tachycardia.

Int J Clin Pract 2004; 58: 807-8.

29. Li L, Cerilli LA, Wick MR.

Inflammatory pseudotumor (myofibroblastic tumor) of the heart.

Ann Diagn Pathol 2002; 6: 116-21.

30. Coffin CM, Watterson J, Priest JR, Dehner LP.

Extrapulmonary inflammatory myofibroblastic tumor (inflammatory pseudo-tumor). A clinic-pathologic and immune-histochemical study of 84 cases.

Am J Surg Pathol 1995; 19: 859-72.

31. Marx GR.

Cardiac tumors.

Heart disease in infants, children, and adolescents: including the fetus and young adult 1995; 2: 1773-86.

32. Skarin A.

Primary cardiac angiosarcoma presenting as a malignant pericardial effusion.

J. Clin. Oncol 1998; 16: 3913-5.

33. Jacabson E.

Two cases of so-called myxofibroma of the heart valves, producing clinical symptoms and congenital vitium.

Annales pediatrici 1943; 161: 1-12.

34. Elderkin RA, Radford DJ.

Primary cardiac tumours in a paediatric population.

J Paediatr Child Health 2002; 38: 173-7.

35. Blondeau P, Soyer R, Piwnica A, Cachefa JP, Dubost C.

Diagnostic and therapeutic problems posed by auricular myxomas.

Ann Chir Thorac Cardio Vasc 1973; 12: 301-6.

36. Conces DJ, Vix VA, Klatte EC.

Gated MR imaging of left atrial myxomas.

Radiology 1986; 156: 445-7.

37. Hansen F, Lyngborg F, Andersen M, Wennevold A.

Right atrial myxomas.

Acta Med. Scand 1969; 86: 165.

38. Saint John Sutton MG, Mercier LA, Giuliani ER, Lie JT.

Atrial myxomas: A review of clinical experience in 40 patients.

Mayo Clin. Proc 1980; 55: 371-6.

39. Arenzana J, Guerra JA, Casero A, Merino J.

A myxoma in the posterior wale of the right atrium.

Rev Clin Esp 1993; 192: 297-8.

40 Mac Allister HA Jr.

Primary tumors of the heart and pericardium.

Pathol. Annals. 1979; 14: 335-55.

41. Mac Allister HA Jr.

Tumors of the heart and pericardium.

Cardiovascular pathology, New York 1983; 917-21.

42. Mc Allister H.A. JR, Fenoglio J.J. JR.

Tumors of the cardiovascular system.

Ed. AFIP, Washington, 1978; 5-20.

43. Molina JE, Edwards JE, Ward HB.

Primary cardiac tumors: experience at the University of Minnesota.

Thorac Cardiovasc Surg 1990; 38: 183-91.

44. Goswami KC, Yusuf A, Anandaraja S, et al.

Clinical and echocardiographic profile of cardiac myxomas.

Indian Heart J Sept-Oct 2003; 55 (5) [Article No. 79].

45. Morrison BJ, Eagle KA.

Left atrial myxomas presenting as a cute respiratory failure.

Chest 1994; 105: 1282-3.

46. Marvasti MA, Obeid AI, Patts JL, Parker FB.

Approach in the management of atrial myxoma with long term follow-up.

Annals Thorac. Surg 1984; 38: 53-8.

47. Pavie A, Escande G, Cham B et al.

Right atrial myxomas: about 3 observations and review of the literature.

Arch Mal Cœur 1981; 74: 265-72.

48. Kyle W. Klarich, Maurice Enrikez-Sarano, George M. Gura, William D, Edwards, A. Jamil Tajik, James B, Seward.

Papillary Fibroelastoma: Echocardiographic Characteristics for Diagnosis and Pathologic Correlation.

JACC 1997; 30: 784-90.

49. Bisel HF, Wróblewski F, LaDue JS.

Incidence and clinical manifestations of cardiac metastases.

JAMA 1953; 153: 712 - 715.

50. Malaret GE, Aliaga P.

Metastatic disease to the heart.

Cancer 1968; 22: 457-66.

51. Young JM, Goldman IR.

Tumor metastasis to the heart.

Circulation 1954; 9: 220-9.

52. GlockY, Herreros J, Arcas R, Mascabuan R, Saidi M, Puel L.

Cardiac myxoma: diagnosis, treatment and late outcome (about an observation of 15 cases).

Heart 1985; 15: 253-62.

53. Gassman HS, Meadows R, Baker LA.

Metastatic tumors of the heart.

Am J Med 1955; 19: 357-65.

54. Seibert KA, Rettenmier CW, Waller BF et al.

Osteogenic sarcoma metastatic to the heart.

Am J Med 1982; 73: 136-41.

55. Scott RW, Garvin CF.

Tumors of the heart and pericardium.

Am Heart J 1939; 17: 431-6.

56. Peters MN, Hall RZ, Cooley DA, Leachman RD, Garcia E.

The clinical syndrome of atrial myxoma.

Jama 1974; 230: 695-700.

57. Kupsky DF, Newman DB, Kumar G, Maleszewski JJ, Edwards WD, Klarich KW. Echocardiographic features of cardiac angiosarcomas: the Mayo Clinic experience (1976-2013). Echocardiography. 2016; 33: 186-92.

58. Engdberding R, Daniel WG, Erbel R, Kasper W, Lestuzzi C.

Diagnosis of heart tumors by transoesophageal echography: a multi-center study in 154 patients. European Cooperative Study Group.

Eur Heart J 1993; 14: 1223-8.

59. Kaplan LJ, Weiman D, Van Decker W, Sokil AB, Whitman GJ.

Infected biatrial myxoma: transoesophageal echocardiography guided surgical resection.

Ann Thorac Surg 1994, 57: 487-9.

60. Bhan A, Mehrotra R, Choudhary SK, et al.

Surgical experience with intracardiac myxomas: long-term follow-up.

Ann Thorac Surg 1998; 66: 810-3.

61. Copeland JG, Valdes-Cruz L, Sahn DJ.

Endomyocardial biopsy with fluoroscopic and two-dimensional echocardiographic guidance: case report of a patient suspected of having multiple cardiac tumors.

Clin Cardiol 1984; 7: 449-52.

62. Salka S, Siegel R, Sagar KB.

Transvenous biopsy of intracardiac tumor under trans-esophageal echocardiographic guidance.

Am Heart J 1993; 125: 1782-4.

63. Applegate PM, Tajik AJ, Ehman RL, Julsrud PR, Miller FA.

Two-dimensional echocardiographic and magnetic resonance imaging observations in massive lipomatous hypertrophy of the atrial septum.

Am J Cardiol 1987; 59: 489-91.

64. Zamorano J, Vilacosta I, Almei AC, San Roman A, Castillo JA.

Contribution of trans oesophageal echocardiography in the assessment of cardiac myxomas.

Rev Esp Cardiol 1994; 47: 17-22.

65. Kuhl H.P, Bucker A, Franke A et al.

Trans-esophageal 3 dimensional echocardiography: in vivo determination of left ventricular mass in comparison with magnetic resonance imaging.

J. Am. Soc. Echocardiography 2000; 13: 205-15.

66. Andrew R.J. Mitchell, Jonathan Timperley, Lucy Hudsmith, Stefan Neubauer, Yaver Bashir.

Intracardiac echocardiography to guide myocardial biopsy of a primary cardiac tumour.

The Europeen society of cardiology 2006; xxx Published by Elsevier Ltd.

67. Aggoun Y, Hunkeler N, Destephen M, Vial Y, Gudinchet F, Calame A et al.

Cardiac rhabdomyomatosis and tuberous sclerosis of Bourneville in the fetus. About 2 cases.

Arch Mal Cœur 1992; 85: 609-13.

68. Godwin JD, Axel L, Adams JR et al.

Computed tomography: A new method for diagnosing tumor of the heart.

Circulation 1981; 63: 448-51.

69. Marazuela M, Garci Merino A, Yebra M et al.

Magnetic resonance imaging and angiography of the brain in embolic left atrial myxoma.

Neuroradiology 1989; 31: 137-9.

70. Grollier G, Lawy E, Khayat A, Foucault JP.

Tumor vasculature in a case of asymptomatic myxoma.

Arch Mal Cœur 1985; 4: 653-6.

71. Van Cleemput J, Daenen W, De Geest H.

Coronary angiography in cardiac myxoma: findings in 19 consecutive cases and review of the literature.

Cathet Cardiovasc Diagn 1993; 29: 217-20.

72. Delisle M.B, Selves J, Alard C et al.

Cardiac sarcoma revealed by blood hypereosinophimia.

Ann. Pathol 1991; 11: 271-4.

73. Kaminskey P, Klein M, Pinelli G, Grasser B, Due M, Villemot JP.

Positive lupus band test in cardiac myxomas.

Lancet 1992; 340: 1100.

74. Saji T, Matsuo N, Shiono N, Yokomuro H, Watanabe Y, Takanashi Y, Komatsu H.

Serum/ tissue interleukin 6 concentrations and constitutional abnormalities in 4 patients with cardiac myxomas.

Kokyu to Junkan 1993; 41: 891-5.

75. Kanda T, Dmeyama S, Sasaki A, Nakazato Y, Morishita Y, Imai S et al.

Interleukin 6 and cardiac myxomas.

The American Journal of Cardiology 1994; 74: 965-7.

76. Kanda T, Nakajima T, Sakamoto H, Suzuki T, Murat K.

An interleukin 6 secreting myxoma in a hypertrophic left ventricle.
Chest 1994; 105: 962-3.

77. Kishimoto T, Hirano T, Kikutani H.

Regulation orifice human B cell differenciation: molecular structure and immunological functions orifice human B cell differenciation factor.

Progress in immunology 1986; 6: 357-67.

78. Bulkey BH, Hutchins GM.

Atrial myxomas: a fifty-year review.

Am Heart Journal 1979; 97: 639-43.

79. Reynen K.
Cardiac myxomas.

N Engl J Med 1995; 333: 1610-7.

80. Monges G, Sudan N, Delpuech F et al.

Myxomas of the heart: an ultrastructural study (about five observations).

Arch. Anat. Cytol. Path 1979; 27: 19-24.

81. Rubin MA, Snell JA, Tazelaar HD, Lack EEL, Austenfeld JL, Azumi N.

Cardiac papillary fibroelastoma: an immunohistochemical investigation and unusual clinical manifestations.

Mod Pathol 1995; 8: 402-7.

82. Yamamoto H, Oda Y, Saito T, Sakamoto A, Miyajima K, Tamiya S, et al.

P53 Mutation and MDM2 amplification in inflammatory myofibroblastic tumours. Histopathology 2003; 42: 431-9.

83. Butany J, Dixit V, Leong S, Daniel L, Mezody M, David T.

Inflammatory myofibroblastic tumor with valvular involvement: a case report and review of the literature.

Cardiovascular Pathology 2007; 16: 359-64.

84. Kelly SJ, Lambie NK, Singh HP.

Inflammatory myofibroblastic tumor of the left ventricle in an older adult.

Ann Thorac Surg 2003; 75: 1971-3.

85. Sherif S. Iskander, Sherif F. Nagueh, Mary L. Ostrowski, and Michael J. Reardon. Growth of a Left Atrial Sarcoma Followed by Resection and Autotransplantation.

Ann Thorac Surg 2005; 79:1771-4.

86. John M. Cho, Gordon K. Danielson, Francisco J. Puga, Joseph A. Dearani, Christopher G. A. McGregor, Henry D. Tazelaar, and Donald J. Hagler.

Surgical Resection of Ventricular Cardiac Fibromas: Early and Late Results.

Ann Thorac Surg 2003; 76:1929-34.

87. Basarici I, Demir I, Yilmaz H, Altekin E.

Obstructive metastatic malignant melanoma of the heart: Imminent pulmonary arterial occlusion caused by right ventricular metastasis with unknown origin of the primary tumor.

Heart and Lung 2006; 35: 351-4.

88. Niels J. Verberkmoes, Suzanne Kats, Ivonne Tan-Go and Jacques P.A.M. Schönberger.

Resection of a lipomatous hypertrophic interatrial septum involving the right ventricle.

Interact CardioVasc Thorac Surg 2007; 6: 654-7.

89. Maryam Esmaeilzadeh, Rozita Jalalian, Majid Maleki, Nader Givtaj, Kambiz Mozaffari, Mozhgan Parsaee.

Cardiac cavernous hemangioma.

Eur J Echocardiography 2007; 8: 487-506.

90. Bic J.F, Frade Schneller O, Marie B et al.

Cardiac angiosarcoma revealed by lung metastases.

Eur. Respir. J 1994; 7: 1194-6.

91. Dulac Y, Plat G, Taktak A, Bassil R, Zabalawi A, Paranon S, Rumeau P, Marcoux M, Acar P.

Large cardiac tumor revealed by ventricular rhythm disturbance in an 18-month-old infant.

Archives of Pediatrics 2006; 13: 1416-9.

92. Garnier P, Michel D, Antoine JC, Solvet P, Gain P, Barral F, Comtet C.

Left atrial myxoma with neurological manifestations: 8 cases.

Revue Neurol 1994; 150: 776-84.

93. Eriksen VH, Baandrup U, Jensen BS.

Total disruption of left atrial myxoma causing a cerebral attack and a saddle embolus in the iliac bifurcation.

Int J Cardiol 1992; 35: 127-9.

94. Zernovicky F, Kubis J, Vrtik L.

Myxoma embolizing into both lower extremities.

Rozhe chir 1994; 73: 127-8.

95. Hashimoto H, Takahashi H, Trijiwara Y, Joh T, Tomino T.

Acute myocardial infarction due to coronary embolisation from left atrial myxoma.

J P N Circ J 1993; 57: 1016-20.

96. Tanabe J, Williams RL, Diethrich EB.

Left atrial myxoma: association with acute coronary embolisation in an 11 years-old boy. Pediatrics 1979; 63: 778-81.

97. Uemura K, Hiramatsu T, Kuzi T, Satoh H, Tomino T.

A case of left atrial myxoma with acute myocardial infarction emergency coronary artery bypass grafting and removal of left atrial myxoma.

Nippon Kyobu Geka Gakkai Zasshi 1993; 41: 1386-9.

98. Taiseer AN, Francis I.

Atrial myxoma producing acute aortic occlusion with anuria and paraplegia: a case study. Vascular Surgery 1986; 277-82.

99. Saitoh H, Kubota H, Takeshita M, Mizuno A, Suzuki M.

Right atrial myxoma with right to left shunt and coronary artery disease.

JPN Circ J 1994; 58: 76-9.

100. Powers JC, Falkoff M, Heinle RA, Nanda NC, Ong L, Weiner RS, Barold SS.

Familial cardiac myxoma: emphasis on usual clinical manifestations.

J. Thorac. Cardiovasc. Surg 1979; 77: 782.

101. Heath D, Mackinnon J.

Pulmonary hypertension due to myxoma of the right atrium.

Am. J. Cardiol 1964; 68: 227-35.

102. Damasio H, Seabra-Gomes R, Da Silva JP, Damasio AR, Lobo Antunes J.

Multiple cerebral aneurysms and cardiac myxoma.

Arch Neurol 1975; 32: 269-70.

103. Loire R, Tabib A.

Histopathological study of cardiac myxoma. About eighty operated cases.

Arch. Anat. Cytol. Pathol. 1991; 39: 5-13.

104. Burton C, Johnston J.

Multiple cerebral aneurysms and cardiac myxomas.

New Engl J Med 1970; 282: 35-6.

105. Price DL, Harris JL, New PEJ, Cante RC.

Cardiac myxoma. A clinicopathologic and angiographic study.

Arch. Neurol. 1970; 23: 558-67.

106. Loeper J, Rouffy J, El Hachimi A, Hammou JC, Chomette G.

Myxoma of the left atrium stimulating diffuse inflammatory arteriopathy.

Ann. Internal Medicine 1970; 121: 559-66.

107. Chen HJ, Liou CW, Chen L.

Metastatic atrial myxoma presenting as intracranial aneurysms with hemorrhage: case report.

Surg Neurol 1993; 40: 61-4.

108. Strauss R, Merliss R.

Primary tumor of the heart.

Arch Pathol 1945; 39: 74.

109. Hiroaki Konishi, Minoru Fukuda, Morito Kato, Yoshio Misawa, and Katsuo Fuse.

Organized Thrombus of the Tricuspid Valve Mimicking Valvular Tumor.

Ann Thorac Surg 2001; 71: 2022-4.

110. Boone SA, Campagna M, Walley VM.

Lambl's excrescences and papillary fibroelastomas: are they different?

Can J Cardiol 1992; 8: 372-6.

111. Semb B. KH, Wexels JC, Vatne K, Bjarnstad PG.

Angiographic and echocardiographic observations in surgical patients with atrial myxoma. Cardiovasc Intervent Radiol 1985; 8: 119-26.

112 Yee HC, Nwosu JE, Lii AD, Velasco M, Millman A.

Echocardiographic features of papillary fibroelastoma and their consequences and management.

Am J Cardiol 1997; 80: 81-4.

113. Muhler EG, Kienast W, Turniski-Harder V, et al.

Arrhythmias in infants and children with primary cardiac tumours.

Eur Heart J 1994; 15: 915-21.

114. Burke A, Tazelaar H, Butany J et al.

Cardiac sarcomas. In: Travis WD, Brambilla E, Mueller-Hermelink HK et al, eds. Pathology and Genetics of Tumours of the Lung, Pleura, Thymus and Heart.

Lyon, France: IARC Press, 2004: 273-81.

115. Botta L, Dell'Amorea A, Pirinib M, D'Andreac A, Mastrorillid M, Mikus P.

Intrapericardial lipoma: successful resection of a giant tumor without cardiopulmonary bypass.

Cardiovascular Pathology 2007; 16: 122-4.

116. Ravikumar E, Pawar N, Gnanamuthu R, Sundar P, Cherian M, Thomas S.

Minimal access approach for surgical management of cardiac tumors.

Ann Thorac Surg. 2000; 70: 1077-9.

117. Jennifer F. Sciuchetti, Fabrizio Corti, Dario Ballabio, Francesco Formica, Angela Aiello, Giovanni Paolini.

Video-assisted thoracic surgical resection of giant cardiac lipoma: A case report. International Journal of Cardiology 2008; 123: 57-8.

118. Attum AA, Johnson GS, Masri Z, Girardet R, Lansing AM.

Malignant clinical behaviour of cardiac myxomas and "myxoid imitators".

Ann Thorac Surg 1987; 44: 217-22.

119. Pezzella AT, Utley JR and Vander Salm TJ.

Operative Approaches to the Left Atrium and Mitral Valve: An Update.

Operative Techniques in Thoracic and cardiovascular surgery 1998; Vd3, No 2: 74-94.

120. Blondeau P.

Primary cardiac tumors-French studies of 533 cases.

Thorac Cardiovasc Surg 1990; 38: 192-5.

121. Jones D, Hill RC, Abbott Jr AE, Gustafson RA, Murray GF.

Unusual location of an atrial myxoma complicated by a secondum atrial septal defect.

Ann Thorac Surg 1993; 55: 1252-3.

122. Jones D, Warden H, Murray G et al.

Biatrial approach to cardiac myxomas: a 30 years clinical experience.

Ann Thorac Surg 1995; 59: 851-6.

123 Kabbani S, Jokhadar M, Meada R, Jamil H.

Atrial myxoma: report of 24 operations using the biatrial approach.

Ann Thorac Surg 1994; 58: 483-8.

124 Indra A.J. Nordstrand, and Robert K.W. Tam.

Minimally Invasive Surgery for Cardiac Myxomas using an Upper Hemi-Sternotomy and Biatrial Septal Approach.

Heart Lung and Circulation 2005; 14: 255-61.

125. Bortolotti U, Maraglino G, Rubino M et al.

Surgical excision of intra cardiac myxomas: a 20-year follow-up.

Ann Thorac Surg 1990; 49: 449-53.

126. Filsoufi F, Fuzellier JF and Fabiani JN.

Surgery for acquired mitral valve lesions (I).

EMC, techniques chirurgicales-Thorax, 42-530, 1998, 12 p.

127. Smith CR.

Septal-superior exposure of the mitral valve. The transplant approach.

J Thorac Cardiovasc Surg 1992; 103: 623-8.

128. Kumar N, Saad E, Prabhakar G, De Vol E, Duran CMG.

Extended TRANS-septal versus conventional left atriotomy: early postoperative study.

Ann Thorac Surg 1995; 60: 426-30.

129. Utley JR, Leyland SA, Nguyenduy T.

Comparison of outcomes with three atrial incisions for mitral valve operations. Right lateral, superior septal, and trans-septal.

J Thorac Cardiovasc Surg 1995; 109: 582-7.

130. Tschirkov A, Michev B et al.

Incidences and surgical aspects of cardiac myxomas in Bulgaria.

Thorac Cardiovasc Surgeon 1990; 38: 196-200.

131. Loire R.

Intracardiac myxomas.

Médicorama 1990; 288.

132. Takach TJ, Reul GJ, Ott DA, Cooley DA.

Primary cardiac tumors in infants and children: immediate and long-term operative results.

Ann Thorac Surg 1996; 62: 559-64.

133. Donald B. Doty, John R. Doty, Bruce B. Reid, and Jeffrey L. Anderson.

Left Atrial Sarcoma: Resection and Repair by Cardiac Autotransplant and In Situ Pericardial Patch.

Ann Thorac Surg 2006; 82: 1514-7.

134. Reardon MJ, DeFelice CA, Sheinbaum R, Baldwin JC.

Cardiac autotransplant for surgical treatment of a malignant neoplasm.

Ann Thorac Surg 1999; 67: 1793-95.

135. Thomas CR Jr, Johnson GW Jr, Stoddard MF, Clifford S.

Primary malignant cardiac tumors: update 1992.

Med Pediatr Oncol 1992; 20: 519-31.

136. Burke A, Cowan D, Virmani R.

Primary sarcomas of the heart.

Cancer 1992; 69: 387-95.

137. Babatasi G, Massetti M, Agostini D et al.

Leiomyosarcomas of the heart and large vessels.

Ann. Cardiol. Angéiol 1998; 47: 451-8.

138. Nakamichi T, Fukada T, Suzuki T et al.

Primary cardiac angiosarcomas: 53 months survival after multidisciplinary therapy.

Ann. Thorac. Surg 1997; 63: 1160-1.

139. Romberg W, Grass M.

Angiosarcoma of the right atrium: local control via low radiation doses and razoxane. Strahlenther.

Oncol 1999; 175: 102-4.

140. Blay J.Y, Bonichon F, Bui B.N et al.

Standards, options and recommendations for the management of adult patients with soft tissue sarcomas.

Arnette Blackwrll 1995; 1: 1-113.

141. Percy R, Perryman R, Amornmarn R et al.

Prolonged survival in a patient with primary angiosarcoma of the heart.

Am. Heart. J 1987; 113: 1228-31.

142. Herrmann M, Shankerman R, Edwards W et al.

Primary cardiac angiosarcoma: a clinicopathologic study of six cases.

J. Thorac. Cardiovasc. Surg 1992; 103: 655-64.

143. Libshitz H.I, Southard M.E.

Complications of radiation therapy: the thorax. Semin.

Roentgenol 1984; 9: 41-9.

144. Das Narla L, Siddiqi NH, Hingsbergen EA.

Inflammatory pseudotumor of the right atrium.

Pediatr Radiol 2001; 31: 351-3.

145. Le Cesne A.

Chemotherapy of metastatic soft tissue sarcomas.
Presse. Méd 1995; 24: 1214-20.

146. Han P, Drachtman R, Amenta P et al.

Successful treatment of a primary cardiac leiomyosarcoma with ifosfamide and etoposide.

J. Pediatric. Hematology/ oncology 1996; 18: 314-7.

147. Lombart-Cussac A, Pivot X, Cotesso G et al.

Adjuvant chemotherapy for primary cardiac sarcomas: the I.G.R experience.

Br. J. Cancer 1998; 78: 1624-28.

148. Shanmugam G.

Primary cardiac sarcoma.

European Journal of Cardio-thoracic Surgery 2006; 29: 925-32.

149. Abu Nassar SG; Parker JC.

Sarcoma Meta-analysis Collaboration.

Adjuvant chemotherapy for localised resectable soft-tissue sarcoma of adults: Meta-analysis of individual data.

Lancet 1997; 350: 1647-54.

150 Nakagawa Y, Ikeda U, Hirose M, et al.

Successful treatment of primary cardiac lymphoma with monoclonal CD20 antibody (rituximab).

Circ J 2004; 68: 172-3.

151. Mayer F, Hermann A, Rudert M, Kinigstreiner M, Horger M, Kanz L, Michael B, Ziemer G, Hartmann J.

Primary Malignant Sarcomas of the Heart and Great Vessels in Adult Patients: A Single-Center Experience.

Oncologist 2007; 12: 1134-42.

152. Hussong JW, Brown M, Perkins SL, et al.

Comparison of DNA ploidy, histology, and immunohistochemical findings with clinical outcome in inflammatory myofibroblastic tumors.

Mod Pathol 1999; 12: 279-86.

153. Ferbend P, Abramson LP, Backer CL, Mavroudis C, Webb CL, Doll JA, et al.

Cardiac plasma cell granulomas: response to oral steroid treatment.

Pediatr Cardiol 2004; 25: 406-10.

154. Pearson PJ, Smithson WA, Driscoll DJ, Banks PM, Ehman RE.

Inoperable plasma cell granuloma of the heart: spontaneous decrease in size during an 11- month period.

Mayo Clin Proc 1988; 63: 1022-5.

155. Meyns B, Vancleemput J, Flameng W, Daenen W.

Surgery for cardiac myxoma. A 20-year experience with long term follow up.

Eur J Cardiothorac Surg 1993; 8: 437-40.

156. Surgimoto T, Ogawa K, Asada T, Mukohara N et al.

Surgical treatment of cardiac myxoma and its complications.

Cardiovasc Surg 1993; 4: 395-8.

157. Castelli E, Ferran V, Octavio de Toledo, Cabbet JM et al.

Cardiac myxomas: surgical treatment, long term results and recurrence.

J Cardiovasc Surg 1993; 34: 49-53.

158. Karnak I, Senocak ME, Ciftci AO, et al.

Inflammatory myofibroblastic tumor in children: diagnosis and treatment.

J Pediatr Surg 2001; 36: 908-12.

159. Roeltgen DP, Weiner G, Patterson LF.

Delayed neurologic complications of left atrial myxomas.

Neurology 1981; 31: 8-13.

160 Donsbeck AV, Ranchere D, Coindre JM, et al.

Primary cardiac sarcomas: an immunohistochemical and grading study with long term follow-up of 24 cases.

Histopathology 1999; 34: 295-304.

161. Mandard A.M, Petiot J.F, Manay J et al.

Prognostic factors in soft tissue sarcomas. A multivariate analysis of 109 cases.

Cancer 1989; 69: 1437-51.

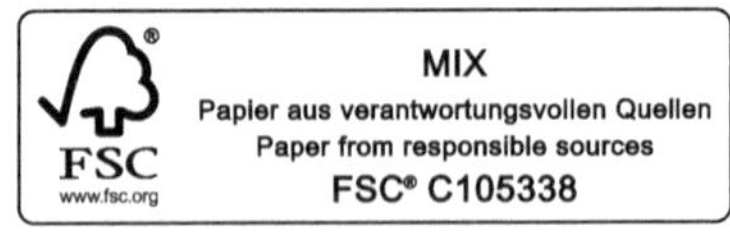

Printed by Books on Demand GmbH, Norderstedt / Germany